FOUNDING THE LIFE DIVINE

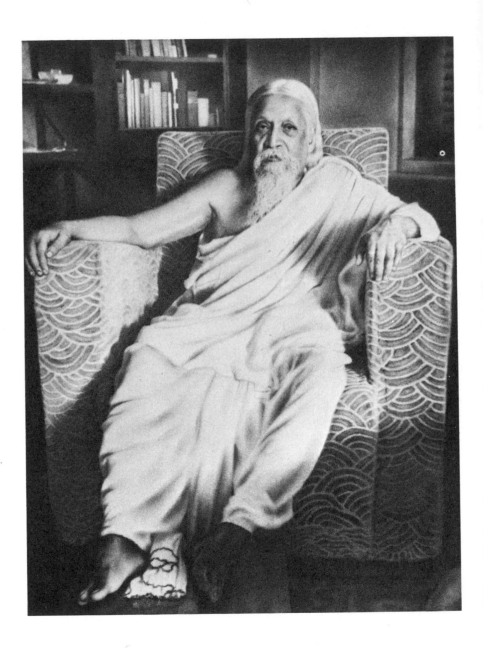

Founding the life divine

An Introduction to the Integral Yoga of Sri Aurobindo

Morwenna Donnelly

The Laughing Man Series of Classic Spiritual Literature

THE DAWN HORSE PRESS
LOWER LAKE, CALIFORNIA

THE DAWN HORSE PRESS
P.O. Box 677
Lower Lake, California 95457

Frontispiece photo by Sri Aurobindo Ashram, courtesy of
Matagiri, Mt. Tremper, N.Y. 12457.

First Dawn Horse Press edition published May, 1976

International Standard Book Number: 0-913922-13-7

Library of Congress Card Catalog Number: 74-24307

Printed in the United States of America

To the guidance and inspiration of a great Master this small book is offered in love and homage

You know the three things on which the realization has to be based:

On a rising to a station above the mind and on the opening out of the cosmic consciousness;
On the psychic opening; and
On the descent of the higher consciousness with its peace, light, force, knowledge, Ananda, etc. into all the planes of the being down to the most physical.

All this has to be done by the working of the Mother's force aided by your aspiration, devotion and surrender.

That is the Path. The rest is a matter of working out of these things for which you have to have faith in the Mother's working.

On Yoga III, *by Sri Aurobindo*

CONTENTS

PART I

APPROACHING THE YOGA

Chapter

8 CONTENTS

CONTENTS

This . . . is the first necessity, that the individual, each individual, shall discover the spirit, the divine reality within him and express that in all his being and living. A divine life must be first and foremost an inner life: for since the outward must be the expression of what is within, there can be no divinity in the outer existence if there is not the divinization of the inner being.

The Life Divine, Vol. II (2), p. 1114.

A general spiritual awakening and aspiration in mankind is indeed the large necessary mot've power, but the effective power must be something greater. There must be a dynamic re-creating of individual manhood in the spiritual type. . . . But spirituality is in its very nature a thing subjective and not mechanical; it is nothing if it is not lived inwardly and if the outward life does not flow out of this inward living. . . . Spiritual truth . . . is of no avail to humanity here, it does not become truth of earth, truth of life until it is lived. The divine perfection is always there above us; but for man to become divine in consciousness and act and to live inwardly and outwardly the divine life is what is meant by spirituality; all lesser meanings given to the word are inadequate fumblings or impostures.

The Human Cycle, pp. 325–26.

The kingdom of God on earth—his kingdom within in men's spirit and therefore, for the one is the material result of the effectivity of the other, his kingdom without in the life of the peoples.

The Human Cycle, p. 323.

Our aim is not . . . to found a religion or a school of philosophy or a school of Yoga, but to create a ground and a way of spiritual growth and experience and a way which will bring down a greater Truth beyond the mind but not inaccessible to the human soul and consciousness. All can pass who are drawn to that Truth, whether they are from India or elsewhere, from the East or from the West. All may find great difficulties in their personal or common human nature; but it is not their physical origin or their racial temperament that can be an insuperable obstacle to their deliverance.

Letters, Vol. IV, p. 55.

The traditions of the past are very great in their own place, in the past, but I do not see why we should merely repeat them and go no farther. In the spiritual development of the consciousness upon earth the great past ought to be followed by a greater future.

Letters, Vol. II, p. 323.

NOTE

Some of the material in this book has already appeared
in reviews and articles on Sri Aurobindo. The chapter
'Divine Source and Divine Meaning' was based on a
lecture given to the London Personalist Group in 1950
on *The Philosophy of Sri Aurobindo*, which he himself
kindly corrected first. The chapter 'Knowledge, Works
and Love' appeared originally, in an extended form, in
The Wind and the Rain (Volume V, Summer 1948) under
the title 'Divine Becoming: the Message of Sri Aurobindo',
and was later reprinted in the *Burning Glass Papers*
(No. 16) and subsequently in India, in *The Advent* and in
Aditi.

I wish to thank most gratefully all the friends who by
their advice and encouragement helped materially in the
writing of this book. To the Head of the Sri Aurobindo
Ashram, Pondicherry, known more widely as 'the Mother',
my warm thanks are also due for her kind permission to
use any quotations I wished from Sri Aurobindo's published works, and to Sri Nolini Kanta Gupta, secretary
of the Ashram, who greatly assisted me by reading this
book in manuscript.

M. D.

PREFACE

IT WOULD be impossible at this close range to his life to assess with completeness the significance of anyone so prodigiously endowed with gifts, both spiritual and intellectual, as Sri Aurobindo. Although his stature as a philosopher and mystic has now received sufficient acclaim in India, Europe and America to establish him as one of the greatest figures of our times, if not, as some believe, the greatest, his real achievement will only be measured adequately by the future, when the goal that he saw humanity must conquer if it is to advance is either realized or has drawn appreciably nearer.

He may be said to occupy a position unique among contemporary philosophers and spiritual thinkers in that he combines in himself two things rarely found together in the same individual: the exposition of an ideal and its attainment. At this transitional period in human history, when modern man, wherever he is allowed to think for himself, is unnerved and bewildered as never before, he speaks therefore with a special authority, holding out to despair a creative alternative which his own life has demonstrated as being no mere empty theory, but capable of realization. "Great in the company of the greatest mystics of all time," as a contemporary thinker has described him, "Aurobindo is the embodiment of a revolution in human life which new knowledge, new powers, new capacities, are creating at this hour." And the same writer[1] goes on to ask, "What is happening to the world because Aurobindo is living in it?" to which he answers, "The world is becoming able to express progressively Unity and Diversity instead of Division, Love instead of Hatred, Truth-Consciousness instead of Falsehood,

[1] The Rev. E. F. F. Hill: *World Review*, October 1949.

17

Freedom instead of Tyranny, Immortality instead of Death; it is becoming progressively that which it is: a movement of the Spirit in itself."

This 'movement of the Spirit' in its unfoldment in the manifested universe forms the core of Sri Aurobindo's theory of evolution. In his major philosophical works he has examined at length the question of the reality and significance of man's existence in the world, basing much of his thought and teaching on the symbolic thinking of the *Vedic* and *Upanishadic* sages and on the *Vedanta* of the *Bhagavad Gīta*. He has insisted that the true character of Indian spirituality is affirmative and life-embracing; that the denial of life, the ideal of a flight to the Absolute which by-passes its difficulties, and all Nihilistic and Quietistic trends, are deviations from the full truth of the ancient vision which pointed, not to an escape from life, but to its fulfilment in and through man.

His interpretation of the nature of reality and the meaning of life convinced him that not only were man and the universe divine in origin, but that a fully divinized life is possible to man in the world and the goal towards which evolution is obscurely labouring—the *raison d'être* of creation.

Sri Aurobindo returned again and again to this theme, expounding and elucidating it with all the resources of a subtle and powerful metaphysical mind which possessed to an outstanding degree the synthetical quality characteristic of the Indian mind at its best. Throughout the principal philosophical studies the multitude of problems connected with this basic certitude are turned in the light of a searching spiritual and intellectual insight and subjected to an exhaustive examination.

Exposition of this kind, however, is perhaps the least part of his astonishing achievement. As a great spiritual Master, himself centred in the ground of the Divine Reality, his object was to bring down into life those powers without which, he believed, man's development could not advance and which (though accessible to him) had not yet been made directly available. It was fundamental to his teaching that until man can achieve an extension of consciousness *beyond* the mental principle which now confines him, he will continue to be trapped by the dilemmas which beset him. He may apply palliatives and effect temporary compromises, but there can be no definitive transformation, no divine life, no kingdom of heaven on earth, unless man can establish his consciousness in a principle to which unity, harmony and truth are native.

In order to take this decisive step forward there must first be an intensive preparation of each individual who aspires to make it. To this spiritual practice Sri Aurobindo gave the name *Purna*, or Integral Yoga.

Though he borrowed from the older systems of Indian Yoga, and particularly from the *Karma Yoga* of the *Bhagavad Gita*, none was comprehensive enough in itself for the object he had in view and Integral Yoga was the result of thirty years' search and spiritual practice. "I think I can say," he wrote of this lifetime of tireless experiment, "that I have been testing day and night for years upon years more scrupulously than any scientist his theory or his method on the physical plane."[1] And again: "Our Yoga is not a retreading of old paths, but a spiritual adventure."[2]

While the great philosophical and metaphysical works of Sri Aurobindo, such as *The Life Divine*, remain outside the scope of many people drawn to the practice of the contemplative life, the reverse may be said of those books in which—mainly in the form of letters to disciples—he outlined his spiritual methods. *The Life Divine* is for those who can (or need) to go by the way of the intellect, for it focusses on the intellectual plane a radiancy of forces above and beyond the resources of the intellect.

[1] *Letters*, Vol. II, p. 69.
[2] *Letters*, Vol. I, p. 28.

Nevertheless, Sri Aurobindo has stated plainly that the fulfilment of the Yoga is not dependent on the intellectual ability of the aspirant. "To see the truth," he said, "does not depend on a big intellect or a small intellect. It depends on being in contact with the Truth and the mind silent and quiet to receive it."[1]

Integral Yoga is intensely relevant to all who feel, not only that new spiritual frontiers stretch out before man which he must reach if he is to fulfil his divine purpose, but that the world is entering a new age where the pattern of spiritual life has still to be discovered and which calls not only for fresh methods, but for an entirely new ideal of human endeavour. Without Yoga there can be no transformed, no divine life, as defined by Sri Aurobindo, for it is only in Yoga that the psychological knowledge exists which is essential to its attainment.

We come up here against a difficulty. In view of the fact that certain Indian Yogas are unsuitable without the direct supervision of a Master—though this unsuitability has been greatly exaggerated[2]—the question naturally

---

[1] *Letters*, Vol. IV, p. 79.

[2] It is worthwhile adding to Sri Aurobindo's statement on the suitability of Yoga for Westerners, the opinion of Sri Krishna Prem, himself a Westerner: "Recently the psychologist Jung, in the course of some sympathetic and interesting comments on a Chinese Taoist book, found occasion to animadvert against those Westerners who practise Eastern yogas. It is quite true that much, probably most, of the so-called yoga practice indulged in by Westerners is foolish and misguided. That is, however, not because it is 'eastern' in origin, but because it is not pursued for the right reason. Yoga is to be undertaken for the sake of Truth itself, for the sake of what the Buddha termed 'unshakable deliverance of heart.' To practise it, as many do, out of curiosity, in search of new sensations, or in order to gain psychic powers is a mistake which is punished with futility, neurosis, or worse. None should seek initiation into the mysteries from unworthy motives, or disaster will surely result. . . . The Path is not a purely Oriental one having, as Jung would say, no roots in a Western psyche, but is something universal to be found in all traditions and fit to be trodden by anyone who has the will to do it." (*The Yoga of the Bhagavad Gita, pp.* xv-xvi.)

arises as to whether Integral Yoga may be safely adopted by the Western aspirant.

Sri Aurobindo's answer is, yes, provided the dedication is sincere and pure. A psychologist of exceptional acuity, his upbringing and education in England gave him, not only an insight into Western temperament, but a deep and critical understanding of Western thought and culture.[1]

He maintained that it was entirely erroneous to believe that Integral Yoga was impossible or unsuitable for non-Oriental natures. "Europeans throughout the centuries," he has written, "have practised with success disciplines which were akin to Oriental Yoga and have followed, too, ways of the inner life which came to them from the East. . . . Especially, since the introduction of Christianity, Europeans have followed its mystic disciplines which were one in essence with those of Asia, however much they may have differed in forms, names, and symbols. . . . It is not the Hindu outlook or the Western that fundamentally matters in Yoga, but the psychic turn and the spiritual urge, and these are the same everywhere."[2]

He saw clearly and dispassionately the strength and weakness of both East and West and how much they could teach each other; in a final analysis, East and West represented to him the two halves of the world psyche and no future could be envisaged without their eventual integration.

[1] Until the age of five Sri Aurobindo spoke only English and Hindustani. When he was seven he was brought by his father, a fervent Anglophil, to England with his two brothers and there given into the care of "an English clergyman and his wife with strict instructions that they should not be allowed to make the acquaintance of any Indian or undergo any Indian influence. These instructions were carried out to the letter and Aurobindo grew up in entire ignorance of India, her people, her religions and her culture." He did not return to India until he was twenty-one. (*Sri Aurobindo on himself and on the Mother.*)

[2] *Letters*, Vol. IV, p. 48 *et seq.*

In clarifying the problems of disciples and in defining the aims and principles of the Yoga, Sri Aurobindo built up a vast body of spiritual lore of a unique kind. Embodying in himself all that was best in the cultures of the East and West—he was a distinguished scholar in Greek and Latin, Italian, French and English, as well as in Sanskrit and Bengali—he can be said to possess a universal character which no other Master of the spiritual life has ever approached in the same way before, and certainly no secular genius. Few teachers, saints, sages or thinkers of modern times have enunciated so revolutionary and joyous a message, or called man so vigorously to acknowledge and *realize* his divine destiny in the world. Few have had a comparable knowledge of history, literature, politics, or been able to meet the arguments of scientific materialism with a more devastating efficiency.

It is with the object therefore of presenting the aims and methods of Integral Yoga and outlining its principles in as simple a way as possible that this book has been written, and to introduce to all who may be searching for its guidance a body of instruction unrivalled in mystical literature.

Integral Yoga has at its heart the *Upanishadic* saying, "The earth is the foundation and all the worlds are upon the earth." The world in which we live is as much in a state of spiritual evolution as we ourselves; because it is divine in origin, perfection is latent in it as it is in us. It follows naturally that, concerned as it is with the earth-consciousness, Integral Yoga turns its face against any withdrawal from life, any form of monastic seclusion, or escape from the challenge of existence in the world. Indeed, Sri Aurobindo has expressly stated that those who cannot face life and its difficulties firmly will never be able to go through the still greater inner difficulties of the Yoga.

It demands of all those courageous enough to stand in

the heat of the battle, the radical transformation of life and personality. Refusing to draw any dividing line between the secular and sacred, it maintains that the field of the divine working is everywhere, and that all work, whether of the hewer of wood or the writer of philosophical treatises, may be made the way of approach to God. To the peoples of these islands, both Celtic and Anglo-Saxon, whose mysticism has always been firmly rooted upon the earth, it should therefore make an especial appeal.

The divine life, in demanding that every aspect of existence be turned towards God, differs only in the *quality* of its activity from life as we understand it. The Yoga asks of those who practise it that they make their lives and work the ground of its action. By striving to liberate the divine reality within the soul and express it, each individual will be able increasingly to bring its creative power into his or her particular corner of existence and, whether this is humble and obscure or powerful and influential, help to open the way for the eventual transformation of life.

"Purified from all that is *aśubha* (evil)," Sri Aurobindo has written in *The Yoga and its Objects*, "transfigured in soul by His touch we have to act in the world as dynamos of that divine electricity and send it thrilling and radiating through mankind, so that wherever one of us stands, hundreds around may become full of His light and force, full of God and full of *ananda* (bliss). Churches, orders, theologies, philosophies have failed to save mankind because they have busied themselves with intellectual creeds, dogmas, rites and institutions . . . as if these could save mankind, and have neglected the one thing needful, the power and purification of the soul. We must go back to the one thing needful, take up again Christ's gospel of the purity and perfection of mankind, Mahomed's gospel of perfect submission, self-surrender and servitude to God,

Chaitanya's gospel of the perfect love and joy of God in man, Ramakrishna's gospel of the unity of all religions and the divinity of God in man, and, gathering all these streams into one mighty river, one purifying and redeeming Ganges, pour it over the death-in-life of a materialistic humanity as Bhagiratha led down the Ganges and flooded with it the ashes of his fathers, so that there may be a resurrection of the soul in mankind and the *Satyayuga* (Age of Truth) for a while return to the world."[1]

With the radical transformation of the individual's nature as its object, Integral Yoga does not pretend to be an easy spiritual way. Sri Aurobindo has described it as the most difficult of all the Yogas. It needs, he warns, an inexhaustible patience and perseverance. The very magnitude of the change it sets before the aspirant makes it more exacting and difficult than any of the older systems. But though its challenge is the challenge of an Everest of the spirit which may not be wholly conquered in our time, it holds out to all who do not believe either in the negation of life as a condition of spiritual liberation, or in a sanctity directed solely towards salvation in the hereafter as the fulfilment of the Divine purpose, but in life more abundantly, an ideal of the spiritual life never expounded before with so wide and diverse a plenitude, or so profound a certainty of its eventual realization.

In this teaching all that is best in Western humanism and Eastern illumination have come together in marriage. To those who set out upon its adventure it demands, likewise, a new combination of qualities. In Sri Aurobindo's own words: "They will adopt in its heart of meaning the inward view of the East which bids man seek the secret of his destiny and salvation within; but also they will accept, though with a different turn given to it, the importance which the West rightly attaches to life and to

[1] P. 57 *et seq.*

the making the best we know and can attain the general life."[1]

With Sri Aurobindo as Teacher, those who venture upon this highest and most difficult, yet joyous, endeavour will surely be able to echo the words of St. Columbcille:

The best guidance from the presence of God
Has been vouchsafed to me.

[1] *The Human Cycle*, p. 330.

FOREWORD

The ascent to the divine Life is the human journey, the
Work of works, the acceptable Sacrifice. This alone is man's
real business in the world and the justification of his
existence, without which he would be only an insect crawl-
ing among other ephemeral insects on a speck of surface
mud and water which has managed to form itself amid the
appalling immensities of the physical universe.

The Life Divine, Chapter IV.

I am glad of my association with this beautiful and
important book, which has been aptly called *Founding
the Life Divine* and which is an exposition of the principles
and aims of Sri Aurobindo's Yoga. For the fundamental
theme of his philosophy and the primary aim of his Yoga
is the Divine Life. The phrase itself reveals the ideal of
a reconciliation and harmony between life and spirituality. The methods for achieving this harmony have been
faithfully and lucidly explained in this book. Because the
exposition is as complete as it can be in a volume of this
size, I shall confine myself to trying to summarize, as far
as possible in his own words, Sri Aurobindo's views, on the
different traditional Yogas of India, which he reviewed as
a preliminary to his exposition of Integral Yoga.

In Sri Aurobindo's view, the processes of Nature and
the methods of Yoga bear a certain correspondence.
Nature is "the cosmic energy and working of God Himself" inspired by an infinite but "minutely selective
wisdom".[1] Yoga, far from being an abnormal activity, is
"in essence a special action or formulation of certain great
powers of Nature".[2] It is a method of self-perfection

[1] *The Synthesis of Yoga, ARYA*, Vol. I, p. 46.
[2] Ibid., p. 37.

27

through the expression of the potentialities latent in the being. These methods bear as much relation to the normal psychological workings of man as do the uses, by applied science, of natural forces like electricity or steam to the ordinary operation of those forces. Likewise, they are formed upon a knowledge developed and confirmed by regular experiment, practical analysis and constant result.

Both *Raja Yoga* and *Hatha Yoga* for example depend on the "perception and experience that the vital forces and functions to which our life is normally subjected and whose ordinary operations seem set and indispensable, can be mastered and the operations changed or suspended with results that would otherwise be impossible and that seem miraculous to those who have not seized the rationale of their process".[1] In less mechanical and more intuitive Yogas, like those of Knowledge and Devotion, this feature of Yoga is not so easily discernible; yet these too start from the use of some principal faculty by ways, and for ends, not contemplated in its everyday, spontaneous working.

Nature herself is engaged in a kind of Yoga in that she is always trying an ever-increasing expression of her potentialities to achieve perfection and to be finally united with the divine reality deeply involved within her. "In man her thinker she for the first time upon this Earth devises self-conscious means and willed arrangements of activities by which this great purpose may be more swiftly and puissantly attained."[2] But Yoga is a means of effecting individual evolution far more rapidly than can the leisurely movements of Nature. A given system of Yoga is thus a selection and compression into more intense forms of the general methods of Nature.

All forms of thought and activity are today being put to a severe test and given a chance of re-birth. Yoga, which Sri Aurobindo thinks is potentially one of the

[1] Ibid., p. 38.
[2] Ibid., p. 37.

dynamic elements of the future life of humanity, is no exception. It is no longer a closed privilege of ascetics and recluses but is coming forward to take its place in human life. Before it can do this adequately, Yoga must rediscover its *raison d'être*, in order to advance to a larger synthesis. Thus reorganized "it will enter more easily and powerfully into the reorganized life of the race".[1]

Before passing to a review of the main Yogas of the past, let us briefly pursue Sri Aurobindo's idea of the correspondence between the processes of Nature and the methods of Yoga.

Evolution, or the self-manifestation of Nature, depends on three successive elements—the evolved, that which is evolving and that which is to be evolved. Physical life has been firmly evolved by Nature; a harmony of matter and life-energy has been accomplished. The former is our foundation and the first condition of our realization; the latter is our means of existence in the material body and the basis of all mental and spiritual activities. A sufficient stability of matter to provide us with a vehicle has been achieved, also a working compromise between the inertia of matter and the active life that lives in and feeds on it.

After bodily life, Nature is evolving mind as her next aim and superior instrument. Man is essentially the thinker, the mental being who leads the life and the body, unlike the animal, which is led by them. But mental life as it is at present evolved is neither a common possession of man nor a finished emergent. The highest expressions of the mind are developed only in individual cases; in the majority they are ill-organized and not easily active. Yet the whole trend of Nature in man is to assure as widely as possible a high general standard of intellectual equipment and capacity. Modern civilization has provided conditions for the development of mental life and these are being universalized. All technological development, spread

[1] Ibid.

of education, progress of the masses—all these should and must result in raising the general standard of the mental level of mankind. This is a great contribution of modern western civilization and though the material and economic values seem to claim all our attention now, the larger impulse will prevail.

It is for the emergence of something truly divine that Nature has taken these steps. What is that goal for the evolution of which the physical existence and life and the mentality of man have been preparing the field? It is here that Yoga intervenes and reveals to us clearly the plan of Nature. All Yogic thought and experience affirm that mind is not the true being of man; it is not the last term of evolution, not an ultimate aim but a means, like the body. Apart from physical and mental being, Yoga recognizes "a third supreme and divine status of 'supramental' being termed the causal body".[1] The characteristic powers of this 'body' are knowledge and bliss. This knowledge is not ordinary mental knowledge but "pure self-existent and self-luminous truth". Bliss too, is not a mere pleasure of the senses but "a self-delight which is the very nature, the very stuff, as it were of a transcendent and infinite existence".[2]

As man is at present constituted, these higher reaches of his being are admittedly super-human; nevertheless, they are states of existence to which his consciousness can open and ascend.

It is clear from the very name of the causal body that it is the source and effective power of all manifestation. It represents the crowning emergent of earthly evolution, even as it is now the secret guide of its process and law. All the levels of our being, physical, mental and emotional, are only deviations from the perfection of divine Being from which they derive. Therefore in Sri Aurobindo's

[1] Ibid., p. 54.
[2] Ibid.

view a perfect liberation does not escape from these things but transforms them. "The fullness of the mental life," he writes, "the suppleness, flexibility and wide capacity of the intellect, the ordered richness of emotion and sensibility are only a passage towards the development of higher life and of more powerful faculties which are yet to manifest and to take possession of the lower instrument, just as the mind itself has so taken possession of the body that the physical being no longer lives only for its own satisfaction but provides the foundation and materials for a superior activity."[1]

It is true that the attraction of the liberation of the truly spiritual element in man is so dazzling that it becomes not only our main but even the sole preoccupation. The persistent ignorances of the mind, the obstinate disturbance of the life-energies, the resistant inertia of the body are so much an obstacle and a burden that the spiritual man feels justified in emancipating his divine soul from its admixture with the other constituents of his total being and nature. But from the point of view of Nature's intention and methods, this ideal is surely a limited aim. For we have seen that "the three steps in Nature are a bodily life which is the basis of our existence here in the material world, a mental life into which we emerge and by which we raise the bodily to higher uses and enlarge it into a greater completeness, and a divine existence which is at once the goal of the other two and returns upon them to liberate them into their highest possibilities. Regarding none of them as beyond our reach or below our nature and the destruction of none of them as essential to the ultimate attainment, we accept this liberation and fulfilment as part at least and a large and important part of the aim of Yoga."[2]

There are three kinds of life man can live both for

[1] Ibid., p. 53.
[2] Ibid., p. 174.

himself and for the community, for Nature herself acts in each of these forms, individually and collectively. He can choose the ordinary material existence; the life of mental activity and development; or that of eternal spiritual felicity. In Sri Aurobindo's system the ideal is neither egoistic assertion of one's own good nor the complete sacrifice of one's self to the community. In relation to the Divine, man's highest ideal is neither to insist on a separate being nor to blot out his existence in the Indefinable. The individual should realize his deepest and highest possibilities and then "pour them out by thought, action and all other means on his surroundings so that the whole race may approach nearer to the attainment of its supreme personalities".[1]

There has always been a double limitation in the spiritual endeavour of mankind. First, the highest spiritual realizations have been for the most part unconnected with the bodily life and the life of the mind. According to Sri Aurobindo, no serious effort has been made till now to make the mind, emotions, actions and physical substance of our being vehicles of the Divine Light and Force. Secondly, those mighty and loving souls who have not remained content with their own realizations, but have mixed with humanity in order to make the great treasures of the Spirit available to all, have not succeeded in establishing more than a noble ethic and a refined religious temperament. A completer and more puissant working of the knowledge and power born of divine realization is what Sri Aurobindo envisages as the aim and goal of his Yoga. According to his vision of things the limited application of the spiritual endeavour of the past is due to the fact that the true source of body, life and mind has not been discovered, with the result that the power that can transform them has not been deployed. For indeed these two are the same and identical reality.

[1] Ibid., p. 174.

Let us now follow Sri Aurobindo in his review of the principles, aims and achievements of the main Yogas of India. He starts by saying that the different natural divisions of the human being and the various utilities founded on them are repeated in the methods of the different Yogas. The heart sublimates its pure emotions to attain bliss. The mind knows its unity with the ineffable reality by converting its ordinary operations to a knowledge beyond itself. The individual self, subjected to the operations of Nature, works in and through them to realize the unconditioned Self.

Yoga is in essence the union of the human consciousness with the divine, "the union of that which has become separated in the play of the universe with its own true self, origin and universality".[1] This union may be affected through all, or any of the levels of the individual being. In the current Indian Yogas we can see an ascending order of progression starting from the body and ending with the direct union of the soul with the Self.

The aim of *Hatha Yoga*, which selects the body and the vital functionings as its means, is the conquest of the life and the body whose balance is the basis of all Nature's activities in man. This balance, sufficient for the normal egoistic life, is not so for the *Hathayogin*, who seeks to create another balance in order to enable the body to sustain an increased flow of vital force, so that there can be a much less fixed and limited action of the universal energy. Fixed posture and breath control are the chief processes of *Hatha Yoga*. It perfects the body, liberates vitality, and by awakening the 'coiled-up serpent' of energy at the base of the spine, opens to the Yogin ranges of consciousness and experience denied to the ordinary human life, while intensifying such powers and faculties as he already possesses.

The achievements of *Hatha Yoga*, though very im-

[1] Ibid., p. 241.

pressive, are won at a very great price. Its detailed and infinitely complicated processes demand complete withdrawal from life so that it cannot be fruitfully utilized for the life of the world. The preservation and perfection of the physical life can be achieved through *Raja Yoga* and the *Tantra* with much less labour and exacting processes. Moreover, there is a risk that the *Hathayogin*, too much preoccupied with abnormal powers, may lose the Divine. The control of nature, rather than spiritual liberation, is looked upon as the hallmark of perfection. Integral Yoga accepts the essential aim of *Hatha Yoga*, that is, the perfecting of the body and the increase and free play of the life-force in it, but it seeks this in order that the body and life can be made perfect instruments of the manifestation of the spirit.

The purpose of *Raja Yoga* is to attain liberation and perfection of the mental being by controlling the emotional and sensational life and mastering the whole range of thought and consciousness. The emotive mind or heart consciousness (*chitta*) in which all the activities originate, is here the main instrument which *Raja Yoga* seeks to quieten and purify. "The preliminary movement of *Raja Yoga* is a careful self-discipline by which good habits of mind are substituted for the lawless movements that indulge the lower nervous being. By the practice of Truth, by renunciation of all forms of egoistic seeking, by abstention from injury to others, by purity, by constant meditation and inclination towards the divine Purusha (soul), who is the true Lord of the mental kingdom, a pure, glad, clear state of mind and heart is established."[1]

While accepting the disciplines of posture and breath-control, *Raja Yoga* rejects the elaborate processes of *Hatha Yoga*. After establishing control over the mind, body and the vital functions, it leads on through a complete 'restriction' of the mental activities to *samadhi*, or

[1] Ibid., p. 244.

Yoga-trance, where the mind by consciously shedding all its activities and springs of action is completely resolved and comes to perfect rest. The soul is thus able to withdraw from its normal identification with the activities of the mind and to enter its true spiritual existence. Secondly, the capacity of force and intense energizing of consciousness is acquired.

Liberation of the soul from the confusions of the mind and the power of self-rule and mastery of the world are achieved through *Raja Yoga*, but its chief limitation is its preoccupation with abnormal states of trance in which the Yogin is absorbed. Here again, in spite of the idea of using released sources of energy for knowledge and mastery of the world, the normal functionings of the mind and physical life are only controlled and quietened but not transformed and transmuted.

The three higher Yogas of Knowledge (*Jnana Yoga*): Devotion (*Bhakti Yoga*): and Work (*Karma Yoga*), attempt what *Raja Yoga* does not and seizing on certain main principles, namely, the intellect, the heart and the will, turns them on the Divine by converting their normal activities. Sri Aurobindo remarks that they do not give the importance bestowed by *Raja Yoga* to the perfection of the mind and body. At the same time each of these Yogas is normally practised in isolation from the others. Both these features are considered by Sri Aurobindo as defects from the standpoint of the Integral Yoga.

The ultimate aim of the Yoga of Knowledge is the realization of the Supreme Self. It proceeds by intellectual inquiry into the nature of the Self to right discrimination between the Self and the not-self. It progressively rejects the false identification with the elements of our phenomenal being, and culminates in the discovery of true identity with the pure and unique Self. "From this point the path, as ordinarily followed, leads to the rejection of the phenomenal worlds from the consciousness as

an illusion and the final emergence without return of the
individual soul in the Supreme."[1]

Sri Aurobindo refuses to accept this fulfilment of the
Yoga of Knowledge as its only result. Not only transcendence by rejection of the cosmic existence, but its conquest
for the Divine can also be the aim. This necessitates, not
only the realization of the Supreme Self in one's own
being, but in all beings, and finally, the realization that
the phenomenal world is a play of the divine consciousness. Indeed, this realization can be extended to include
the conversion of all forms of knowledge into activities
of the divine consciousness. It is conceivable that this
might well lead to the spiritualization of the human intellect and to the "justification of the cosmic travail of
knowledge in humanity".[1]

The dedication of all human activity to the supreme
Will is what the Yoga of Works seeks. By giving up all
egoistic aim in our works and all action for any interest
or worldly result, the mind and will are purified and there
is a clear perception of the cosmic Energy as their ruler.
The Yoga demands the surrender of all works and their
result to the supreme Will and cosmic Energy. The soul
is liberated by these means from its bondage to appear-
ances and to the reaction of phenomenal activities. But
here again the ultimate fulfilment is "liberation from
phenomenal existence and a departure into the Supreme".[2]
Sri Aurobindo says that the perceptions underlying *Karma
Yoga* can lead to the spiritualization of human will and
activity and "to the justification of the cosmic labour
towards freedom, power and perfection in the human
being".[2]

Looking upon the Supreme as the divine Lover and
enjoyer of the universe, the Yoga of Devotion seeks the
enjoyment of the supreme Love and Bliss. This Yoga

[1] Ibid., p. 247.
[2] Ibid., p. 249.

utilizes all human relations into which emotion enters, not
in the ordinary unpurified worldly sense, but by applying
to them the delight of the All-Loving. This also culminates
in the total absorption of the devotee in the bosom of the
Beloved, away from the world's existence; though again,
this need not be the inevitable result. In fact it is provided in the Yoga itself that the relation of love between
the Divine and the devotee may be extended to all living
beings. Sri Aurobindo feels that this Yoga may be applied
to the spiritualization of the whole range of human
emotion and be the "justification of the cosmic labour
towards love and joy in our humanity".[1]

Love and Knowledge and Works need not be exclusive.
Perfect intimacy with the Beloved will bring perfect knowledge of him and divine service; knowledge should lead to
love and the acceptance of works; dedicated works pave
the way to love of the Master of Works, and knowledge
of His ways and His being. "It is in this triple path that
we come most readily to the absolute knowledge, love
and service of the One in all beings and in Its entire
manifestation."[2]

There is a Yoga in India, the *Tantra*, which though not
a conscious synthesis of all the Yogas is yet of a synthetical
turn. The central principle of the *Tantra* is expressly
different from that of the *Vedic* methods of Yoga. In the
latter the soul (*purusha*) is the Lord and the chief method
is knowledge, either by the mind, heart or will. In the
Tantra it is *prakriti*, the nature-soul and Creatrix of the
Universe, who is the Mistress of the Yoga. The *Tantric*
learns the secret methods—the *Tantra*—of the Will-in-
Power to realize his aim in Yoga—mastery, perfection,
liberation and beatitude. In actual practice, however,
partial knowledge of the secret and occult methods of
Nature without sufficient purity of motive and spiritual

[1] Ibid., p. 248.
[2] Ibid., p. 249.

intention, and a tendency to encourage satisfaction of the normal hungers and passions of an unregenerate nature under the garb of spiritual practice, led to serious abuses. This is responsible for the enlightened mind's abhorrence of *Tantra*. It should, however, be made clear that the abuses of a degenerate Tantra must not make us blind to the great merits and achievements of the original and essential *Tantra*.

The limitations of the Yogas very briefly reviewed above, are that they all fix their attention on a realization beyond the cosmos and none to the world and world-values. Also they tend to emphasize the individual's spiritual life and do not envisage any collective spiritual evolution—which, of course, they cannot do, being concerned with supra-cosmic aims. The *Tantra*, more than any of the other Yogas studied above, accepts both the static and dynamic, the transcendent and the cosmic aspects of the Divine equally in its philosophy. But here again, Sri Aurobindo feels, there is too little stress on the soul's divine potentialities, "a haste of insistence on the escape into super-conscience".[1]

It may be worth while at this point to mention briefly Sri Aurobindo's views on the spiritual goals of Buddhism and Christianity. In Buddhism the aim of liberation from suffering and rebirth, with its quintessential experience in a supra-cosmic spiritual realization, is again a limitation from the point of view of the Integral Yoga, which accepts life and the world as the ground of a Divine realization and does not therefore seek to get away from them. "The Christian ideal," he writes, "aims at the attainment of a celestial existence beyond the earth's existence (beyond this single earth life, for reincarnation is not admitted) which is only a vale of sorrows and a passing ordeal."[2] It lacks the realization of perfect identity between the indi-

[1] *The Problem of Rebirth*, p. 51.
[2] *Letters of Sri Aurobindo*, Vol. IV, p. 36.

vidual, the universal and the transcendent Divine, and though it envisages the Kingdom of Heaven on Earth, this is, in Sri Aurobindo's view, only an ethical ideal and has not either the knowledge or the power necessary for the complete transformation of life, as he understands it. Christianity, he says, "has no higher spiritual or psychological knowledge behind it and ignores the foundation of human character and the source of the difficulty—the duality of mind, life and body".[1]

Sri Aurobindo considers therefore that for the purpose of founding a new life on the earth, resultant on the further evolution of man's consciousness, the methods and aims of the older Yogas are incomplete and inadequate.

It is not, however, by combining *en bloc* the different Yogas, nor by their successive practice (if that were possible in one human life) that we can get an Integral Yoga. A common central principle and some fundamental dynamic force which is the secret power of the different Yogas and therefore capable of organizing their aims and utilities, must be seized upon. That principle, in Sri Aurobindo's view, is the *Vijñāna*, the Supermind, which is the Divine's own knowledge of Himself and His own native power of acting. It is this Supermind which the Yoga of Sri Aurobindo aspires to establish in humanity as its normal, organized principle and power of consciousness.

Until now, even the most complete spiritual realization has missed some aspect of the integral Truth and as a consequence, the application of spirituality to life, when at all attempted, has been ineffective or effective only to a limited extent. The embodiment of the Supramental in humanity would lead, not only to a realization of the Divine of the utmost plenitude, but to the possession of that self-effectuating Truth which is the source and power of all creation and the as-yet veiled guide of all the basic

[1] Ibid., Vol. I, p. 39.

aspirations of humanity. Its organization in a number of
people thus promises to usher in a new kind and rhythm
of collective life which will consummate all Nature's
endeavour at self-perfection. For the aim of Integral Yoga
is to "re-unite God and Nature in a liberated and perfected
human life" and its method "not only to permit but
favour the harmony of our inner and outer activities and
experiences in the divine consummation of both".[1]

How this high and comprehensive aim can be achieved,
Sri Aurobindo has shown most lucidly and with great
power in his voluminous writings. In spite of being very
clearly written, Sri Aurobindo's own books are not easy to
approach by people who have no background of spiritual
Philosophy or Yoga. Miss Donnelly's book fulfils a long-
felt want for an authentic, faithful and eminently readable
introduction to Sri Aurobindo's Yoga. All that is of essential value is competently dealt with in this sympathetic
book. People interested in finding a dynamic way to self-
discovery and integral God-realization, and in the application in life of the highest and completest Knowledge
and Power, will find that way described here with felicity
and inspiration. They have every reason to be grateful to
the author for placing in their hands a most useful manual
of the methods of the Integral Yoga, the potent means of
'Founding the Life Divine'.

A. BASU, M.A.

*Spalding Lecturer in Indian Philosophy and Religion,
Durham Colleges in the University of Durham. Member,
Committee of Experts on Translation of Representative
Works, International Council for Philosophic and
Humanistic Studies, Paris.*

---

[1] *The Synthesis of Yoga.* Arya, Vol. I, p. 16.

PART I

Approaching the Yoga

CHAPTER I

DIVINE SOURCE AND DIVINE MEANING

I am concerned with the earth consciousness, not with worlds beyond for their own sake; it is terrestrial realization that I seek and not a flight to distant summits. All other Yogas regard life as an illusion or a passing phase: the supramental (i.e. Integral) Yoga alone regards it as a thing created by the Divine for a progressive manifestation and takes fulfilment of the life and body for its object.
Letters, Vol. III, p. 327.

This Yoga accepts the value of cosmic existence and holds it to be a reality; its object is to enter into a higher Truth-Consciousness . . . in which action and creation are the expression not of ignorance and imperfection, but of the Truth. . . . But for that, surrender of the mortal mind, life and body to that Higher Consciousness is indispensable. . . . Only those who can accept the call to such a change should enter into this Yoga. *Letters*, Vol. I, p. 57.

The way of Yoga followed here has a different purpose from others—its aim is not only to rise out of the ordinary ignorant world-consciousness into the divine consciousness, but to bring the supramental power of that divine consciousness down into the ignorance of mind, life and body, to transform them, to manifest the Divine here and create a divine life in Matter. *Lights on Yoga*, p. 1.

To PLUNGE deeply into the metaphysical foundations of Integral Yoga would confuse the aim of this book, which is to present the principles of the Yoga as simply as possible. It is not essential to understand the metaphysical system behind the Yoga in the profound sense in which it is expounded in *The Life Divine*. Nevertheless,

43

the Yoga is finely geared to its metaphysic—indeed, it springs from it—and it is certainly helpful to have some idea of the conception of God, man and cosmos upon which it is based.[1]

The foundation of the Yoga is the concept: all that is, is God; beside Him nothing else exists. He is not only the basis of creation, One and Indivisible, the supporting energy of all phenomenal existence, who gives Himself equally to all existences. He is also the Transcendent Divine, beyond all multiplicity or oneness, movement or motionlessness—those terms by which we try to image to ourselves His infinity.

For when we have realized God as the Supreme Being, the basis and support of creation and immanent in all things from the star to the stone, from man to the amoeba, we know that as Transcendent Divine He exceeds all that we can attribute to Him and that in His pure and absolute Existence He is beyond anything we can conceive through His manifested or unmanifested Presence.

If all that is, is God, then everything that exists, whether it is ourselves or the created world we see around us in all its myriad variety of inorganic, organic and animal forms, is one existence. 'The Many are the One' as the great classic statement of the ancient Seers expressed it. In its plunge into material life the manifested being of man has lost this knowledge of the unity of all things and sees itself and all others as separate existences. Even when it has caught a reflection of the Divine Being in the world, it still does not know that He is also its highest Self. To

---

[1] Inability to grasp this kind of intellectual exposition should, however, never be allowed to become a bar to the practice of the Yoga. The simplest mind may find through devotion and perfect surrender other ways of entering the Divine mystery. Sri Aurobindo has observed on this point: "I have seen comparatively uneducated people expressing higher knowledge with an astonishing fullness and depth and accuracy which the stumbling movements of their brain could never have allowed one to suppose possible." (*Letters*, Vol. IV, p. 87.)

know God in all things, indivisible though apparently divided into many existences, is therefore an indispensable step, enjoined by all systems of Yoga, towards that truth of inner knowledge and realization which is the final goal.

This "One indivisible that is pure existence", as the *Upanishad* expresses it, is ultimate, or fundamental, Reality. The qualities of this Pure Existence are Consciousness and Force, by which it pours itself into material creation—still, as the Gita tells us, "indivisible, but as if divided in beings". This Conscious-Force of the Divine Being, as we have already said, is in all phenomenal existence.

In the thinking being it strives, as the soul, through self-realization to recover the bliss and infinite consciousness of its divine origin. This self-realization is the divine goal; the apotheosis of spiritual becoming, in which the apparently fragmented consciousness of the individual becomes one with its source. On its attainment the divine life is founded.

Therefore, when we speak of God as 'transcendent' and 'immanent' we are stating the distinction—but not forcing it into an opposition—between Pure Being and *becoming*. This power of Pure Being to create forms—to become the manifested world of which we are a part—which Sri Aurobindo calls Conscious-Force, we in the West might more crudely define as Energy.

Spirit and matter, then, are not opposing principles, but different aspects of the One Being. But this Conscious-Force which throws itself out into manifestation has a dual nature of being at rest or in motion, dynamic or passive. There is not a moment when potentially it is not, for it is eternally free to express itself either in world-play or repose.

The question may well be asked: Why should the One, who is all bliss, all joy, all perfection, all truth, desire to

become involved in the labour of creation and in all the
suffering, anguish, ignorance and division which seem to
characterize material existence? From delight, Sri Aurobindo returns. "Delight is existence, Delight is the secret
of creation, Delight is the root of birth, Delight is the
cause of remaining in existence, Delight is the end of
birth and that into which creation ceases."[1] "For who
could live or breathe if there were not this delight of
existence as the ether in which we dwell?" asks the
Taittiriya Upanishad, and again, "From Delight all these
beings are born, by Delight they exist and grow, to
Delight they return."

We may see creation, then, as a movement of ascent
and descent, "a movement between two involutions,
Spirit in which all is involved and out of which all evolves
downward to the other pole of Matter, Matter in which
also all is involved and out of which all evolves upwards
to the other pole of Spirit".[2]

Without going deeply into the subtle metaphysical
reasoning which refines these statements regarding the
nature and operation of the Divine, we must examine
briefly one further point if we are to understand fully the
aim of Integral Yoga.

Evolution, as Sri Aurobindo sees it, is an unfolding of
the divine potentialities inherent in matter from the most
obscure and insentient beginnings to a full flowering and
"luminous consummation in Spirit", for the subconscient
as well as the superconscient contains this life of the All.
In every stage of evolution in which it has been involved
in material existence, the Divine Consciousness has
laboured to unfold into ever higher and more perfect instruments of expression. The first great emergence took
place with the appearance of organic life; the second, with
the emergence of vital or animal life; the third with man,

[1] *The Life Divine*, Vol. I, p. 121.
[2] Ibid., p. 154.

who was able to embody in Mind the highest level to which consciousness had yet attained in its upward ascent.

But, asks Sri Aurobindo, can we believe that Mind is the high-water mark of this Consciousness in evolution? Is it audacious to suppose that a higher level awaits our attainment when we consider the enormous advances that were made by the evolution of the plant from inorganic matter and then in the appearance of animal life and of man? His answer is, no: not only are we justified in looking forward to a further ascent when we examine the past miraculous upward evolution of life; our speculations are also justified when we examine the processes by which the Divine creates the cosmos.

Here we must go back for a moment to the Conscious-Force which Sri Aurobindo defines as the power put forth by Pure Being to create the phenomenal universe. Between the Supreme Existence of God and 'the flux of the Many' with all its myriad forms of life, there is an intermediary principle which Sri Aurobindo calls the Super-mind,[1] or Truth-Consciousness.

The most abstruse reaches of Sri Aurobindo's thought are concerned with the nature and operation of the Supramental and it would be outside our province to attempt to follow them here, quite apart from the difficulties in the way of interpreting in the terms of the intellect a realm apparently so contradictory to it in essence and activity.

Put as simply as possible, the Truth-Consciousness or

[1] "The sun in the Yoga is the symbol of the Supermind and the Supermind is the first power of the Supreme which one meets across the border where the experience of spiritualized mind ceases and the unmodified divine Consciousness begins the domain of the supreme Nature, *Para Prakriti*. It is that Light of which the Vedic mystics got a glimpse and it is the opposite of the intervening darkness of the Christian mystics, for the Supermind is all light and no darkness. . . . If we follow the line leading to the Supermind, it is an increasing affirmation rather than an increasing negation through which we move." (*Letters*, Vol II, p. 37.)

48   FOUNDING THE LIFE DIVINE

Supermind would seem to be an intermediate functioning
of consciousness between the Pure Being of God and the
inferior functioning of consciousness represented by Mind,
"which can only know by separation and distinction and
has at the most a vague and secondary apprehension of
unity and infinity—for though it can synthetize its
divisions, it cannot arrive at a true totality".[1] We can
imagine it as a movement of God out of His primal purity
which creates the cosmos.

Supermind is not the absolute self-existence of the
Supreme Being, but it is His nature and the operation of
His self-ordering in the universe.

This principle lies at the summit of our being. To dwell
permanently in it is the consummation of the spiritual
man. If we could re-enter its domain we should stand, as
it were, in an instantaneous relation with Truth. Instead
of feeling our way clumsily towards it by methods which
can never embrace it, we should stand within it, and
because we were one with the originating source of all that
is, we should *know* with an absolute truth of knowledge.[2]

Only by returning to the source of knowledge, Sri
Aurobindo maintains, can man have any complete understanding of the mysteries of existence, learn to live in
harmony with himself and others and bring into life a
force capable of transforming it at root, and not one
(like the moral and humanistic) that merely manipulates
certain aspects of it.

But though individuals may rise into higher states of
consciousness that receive the supramental light, to live
and act from this divine principle "is a victory that has
not yet been made humanly possible".[3] Could the conditions for the descent of this power into the earth con-

[1] *The Life Divine*, Vol. I, p. 150.
[2] This realization of being one with the source of Truth is called by
Sri Aurobindo *knowledge by identity*.
[3] *The Life Divine*, Vol. I, p. 148.

sciousness once be established, in however small a degree, Sri Aurobindo knew that a step forward in human evolution of the most decisive magnitude would be accomplished, and it was to this work that latterly he devoted his life.[1]

Between the Supermind and human mentality there is an intermediary principle to which Sri Aurobindo gives the name Overmind. This principle represents a much higher range of consciousness than the human mind, being "a screen of dissimiliar similarity through which Supermind can act directly on an Ignorance whose darkness could not bear or receive the impact of a supreme Light".[2] Spontaneous knowledge—intuition, inspiration and the like—come to us as messengers from this subliminal range

[1] Though no other thinker or mystic has written at such great length and in so detailed a manner of this Supramental level of consciousness, its existence and eventual embodiment in man appears to have been known for many centuries, at least to Mahayana Buddhism. There seem to be close resemblances between the Fifth Element, Ether, in its primal form, "symbolized as 'the green light-path of the Wisdom of Perfected Actions'" and the Dhyani Buddha Vairochana, and the Supermind. In the Fifth Element esoteric Buddhism symbolizes "a transcendental consciousness higher than the normal consciousness in mankind, and as yet normally undeveloped", believing it to be "destined to become the active consciousness of the humanity of the Fifth Round. . . . In place of faith or mere belief, Man will then possess Knowledge, will come to know himself in the sense implied by the Mysteries of ancient Greece . . . and this will come as a normal process of human evolution . . . (This) supramundane Buddha (or *Bodhic*) consciousness has not been developed in the ordinary humanity." (*The Tibetan Book of the Dead*, pp. 9-16. W. Y. Evans-Wentz.) Sri Aurobindo has stated that both in the Vedas and the Upanishads the Supermind is mentioned, and in *The Riddle of this World* (p. 2) writes: "The Vedic Rishis never attained to the Supermind for the earth or perhaps did not even make the attempt. They tried to rise individually to the Supramental plane, but they did not bring it down and make it a permanent part of the earth-consciousness. Even there are verses of the Upanishads in which it is hinted that it is impossible to pass through the gates of the Sun (the symbol of the Supermind) and yet retain an earthly body. It was because of this failure that the spiritual effort of India culminated in Mayavada."
[2] *The Life Divine*, Vol. I, p. 335.

of consciousness, but though knowledge assumes the nature of thought in the Overmind it has a different character from the processes of thought to which we are accustomed.

The characteristic of Mind, or mental life, as defined by Sri Aurobindo, is that it imagines itself as separate; its powers are those of delimitation and formal definition, analysis, division, and discrimination. These powers Mind carries into all its perceptual and creative thought. Being itself only a partial working of consciousness it can no more know the whole, of which it is a limited and distant derivative, than it can know the essence of the thing it scrutinizes.

Mind is therefore the centre of the Ignorance, particularly our self-ignorance, and on it all our errors depend; all those limitations from which our suffering, division and exile from truth proceed. Yet this ignorance is not absolute falsehood. It is distortion of Truth in which Mind has lost the sense of unity with God and all created forms and exalts its native power of division into an absolute. By its very nature, being a limited power of consciousness to which wholeness, harmony and unity are not native, Mind must remain impotent to solve those problems of our existence, both as creatures striving to live in the Divine Light and as members of a world community, which have sprung directly from its own inadequacy as an instrument.

It is only by striving to rise into a principle to which Truth is native and not held in a derivative status, and where unity and harmony are the spontaneous elements, that humanity can overcome the barriers behind which the mental principle has imprisoned it and discover that life of infinite diversity, founded on an absolute unity, which characterizes the divine life.

It will be seen from the foregoing that Sri Aurobindo is concerned with something far more comprehensive than individual salvation. The preparation of the individual for

eternal life beyond the world, for a bliss and perfection
only obtainable in its plenitude hereafter; the conception
of the world itself as a vale of tears from which the soul
must hasten to escape into the bosom of the Infinite, the
miseries of which the spiritually-minded man may allevi-
ate but can never hope radically to alter, were, he maintained, the goals held out with varying emphasis by all
the great religions.[1]

He firmly stated the fundamental divergence from
these aims of his own ideal: "It (Integral Yoga) aims not
at a departure out of world and life into Heaven and
Nirvana, but at a change of life and existence, not as
something subordinate or incidental, *but as a distinct and
central object*. . . . The object sought after is not an individual achievement of divine realization for the sake of
the individual, but something to be gained for the earth-
consciousness here, a cosmic, not solely a supra-cosmic
achievement."[2] Again, "the Yoga we practise, is not for
ourselves alone, but for the Divine; its aim is to work out
the will of the Divine in the world, to effect a spiritual
transformation and *to bring down a divine nature and a
divine life into the mental, vital and physical nature and life
of humanity*. Its object is not physical *mukti* (spiritual
liberation) although mukti is a necessary condition of the
Yoga, but the liberation and transformation of the human
being."[3]

This distinctive aim of Sri Aurobindo's teaching cannot
be emphasized too much. It is far more extensive than
that of any other system of Yoga and sets before humanity
an endeavour more arduous than any enunciated before
by those great spiritual Teachers of the world of whom we

[1] The essentially world-renouncing, world-negating attitude of
Christianity is well summarized by Prof. Radhakrishnan in his *Eastern
Religions and Western Thought*, p. 68 passim.
[2] *Letters*, Vol. I, pp. 26-7. The italics are mine.
[3] *The Yoga and its Objects*, pp. 1-2. The italics are mine.

possess records. Not to grasp this most essential principle of his teaching is to miss his whole distinctive significance as a thinker and teacher.

The idea that the world and man together were slowly evolving towards a perfect flowering in time was one of the deepest convictions of his spiritual philosophy and one that he believed to be supported by his reading of the intricate processes of evolution.

He saw the labour of life, first in the plant, then in the animal, and finally in man as "a progressive series for the unfolding of the Spirit" and one of "supreme significance",[1] and he expounded his reading of this riddle of existence with all the insight, illumination and acute reasoning at his command.

To believe that man, as a mental being, was the apotheosis of creation, or that matter held no higher evolutionary potentialities within it was, he maintained, not only wilfully to misread the evidence, but to circumscribe the divine purpose in the manifested universe and to offer humanity no escape from its dilemmas.

"What is around us," he wrote in *The Problem of Rebirth*, "is the constant process of the unfolding (of the spiritual evolution) in its universal aspect; the past terms are there contained in it, fulfilled, overpassed by us, but in general and various types still repeated as a support and background; the present terms are there not as an unprofitable recurrence, but in active pregnant gestation of all that is yet to be unfolded by the spirit, no irrational decimal recurrence helplessly repeating for ever its figures, but an expanding series of powers of the Infinite. What is in front of us is the greater potentialities, the steps yet unclimbed, the intended mightier manifestations."[2] In short, the very purpose of our existence here is to be the means of the spirit's upward self-unfolding.

[1] *The Problem of Rebirth*, p. 52.
[2] Ibid., p. 53.

CHAPTER II

THE INDIVIDUAL CENTRE

The supreme Self is one, but the souls of the Self are many. *The Life Divine:* passim.

The one infinitely variable Spirit in things carries all of himself into each form of his omnipresence; the self, the Being is at once unique in each, common in our collectivities and one in all beings. God moves in many ways at once in his own indivisible unity.

The Problem of Rebirth, p. 60.

The Divine is always in the inner heart and does not leave it. *Letters,* Vol. IV, p. 178.

The Divine is . . . the Person beyond all persons.
Letters, Vol. I, p. 83.

THE Supreme Being is the source of all manifested existence and the purpose of this existence is that it should grow increasingly in consciousness until it becomes wholly transformed, even into the depths of its most material densities. Man, as the highest point to which the evolving consciousness in matter has yet attained, is the spearhead of this ascent. Therefore, before approaching the practice of the Yoga we must understand the conception of the person—as a centre of the Divine spirit in the world—upon which it is based.

Like all the spiritual disciplines of the East, Integral Yoga is founded on a subtle metaphysical psychology,[1] sometimes called in the West *depth psychology,* and it is

---

[1] The term metaphysical is used here in order to distinguish this system of psychology, based on exacting introspective analysis and observation—in short, on a different method of obtaining knowledge—from the empirical psychologies of the West, based on objective analysis and experiment.

important to understand exactly what Sri Aurobindo means when he uses such terms as vital, mental, or psychic being: soul, self, spirit, ego. Not to understand the precise nature of these distinctions is to end in confusion.

The individual being consists of the highest Self, or Spirit;[1] the soul and psychic being; the mental and vital sheaths[2] (or bodies) which enclose the physical body, and, in all but the liberated man, the egoistic self. All these, with the exception of the ego, are fundamentally projections of the Self, variously organized to support its manifestation in the material world.

The Self is realized, in Sri Aurobindo's words, "as the true being of the individual, but also more widely as the *same being* in all and as the Self in the cosmos". It remains above the manifestation, "pure and stainless, unaffected by the stains of life, by desire and ego and ignorance".[3] In the experience of the Yoga, he adds, it is "an essence one with the Divine or at least it is a portion of the Divine

[1] The Atman. Sri Aurobindo's conception of the Atman or Self is based on that of the Upanishads, but the various Indian schools of thought differ considerably in their views on this subject. The Upanishadic conception of the Atman is well defined by Professor Jadunath Sinha in his book *Indian Psychology Perception* (pp. 245–47). Briefly summarized it is as follows: The Atman is one with the Absolute; it is absolutely unconditioned; it is indefinable by speech and unattainable by the outer or inner senses; it is spaceless, timeless and causeless. It is the ultimate reality, the noumenon, beyond duality and distinction, so that it cannot be an object of knowledge. But though it is absolutely unknowable as the unconditioned Brahman, it is not so as man's inner self, hidden in the heart, where it can be apprehended by yogis or seers through meditation and concentration.

The criticism, so often heard from Christian thinkers, that Hinduism and Buddhism only penetrate to union with the ground of being, is the result of a gross ignorance of the higher metaphysical teachings of these two great spiritual systems.

[2] Strictly speaking, the *ādhāra*, or containing system, is composed of five sheaths, physical, vital, mental, supramental and spiritual being, but in the early stages of the Yoga it is only necessary to understand the working of the first three.

[3] *Letters*, Vol. I, p. 158.

and has all the Divine potentialities".[1] The Self presides over the various life-experiences of the individualized consciousness, but it does not become in any way involved with them, being prior to the evolution and in its highest relation above the individual and the cosmos and one with the Supreme Divine Being.

The soul is an aspect of the Self, "a spark of the Divine . . . which comes down into the manifestation to support its evolution in the material world. . . . This spark is there in all living beings from the lowest to the highest."[2] The psychic being[3] is formed by the soul to support the mind, vital sheath, and body, but is at first veiled by these things and only as it grows becomes capable of coming forward and dominating them. To grow aware of the psychic being, and to bring it forward so that it controls all the levels of the individual, is one of the principal movements of the Yoga. It may be described as the most outlying region of the soul—that part of it with which we may most easily establish contact.

Screening these psychic powers with their divine potentialities is the ego-personality, in which the division of consciousness, the separative, illusory powers of the Mind, are at their strongest. Most people are entirely dominated by this ego—sometimes called the desire-soul —and have no perception of any deeper part of their being. The ego is built up by Nature in the process of evolution. It is a nexus of imperfect consciousness and imperfect knowledge gathered together in the being's push out of the Ignorance. Sri Aurobindo defines it also as a sense which makes man identify himself with the creation that Nature has made of him and with the varying mind, life and body she has constructed.

[1] *Letters*, Vol. I, p. 159.
[2] Ibid., p. 144.
[3] Sri Aurobindo uses the word 'psychic' as referring to the soul, not in the debased modern sense of spiritistic phenomena.

The individual psychic being has to withdraw itself from outward concentration in the ego, with its restless, ephemeral desires and ambitions, it subjective constructions of pain and pleasure, and, wholly possessing itself and its instruments of body and mind, grow fully into union with the Self.

The doctrine of the subtle bodies[1] is an ancient concept of Hindu medicine and psychology, and Sri Aurobindo, when he is speaking of these bodies or sheaths, always assumes a familiarity in his reader with the basic teachings concerning their psychological action and nowhere describes them in general outline, though he has much to say about their specific working.

Scientific research into the nature of the subtle sheaths and of their ultra sonic rates of vibration has made progress in the West in recent years, and the following passage gives a simple and easily understandable description of their function: "Its (the etheric body's) chief activities are two: (i) to act as a subtle matrix for all physiological changes, as the organizer wherein the pattern of the new structure lies, as a vital centre whence directive energies are variously distributed through the more mechanical chemical components of blood, organs and tissue; and (ii) to act as a bridge mechanism especially adapted to link the forces of mind, feeling and will, characteristic of each soul, to its body. A 'live' body possesses such a bridge mechanism and vital matrix. In a dead body the bridge has been broken."[2] The subtle bodies possess seven main centres, called in the East *chakras*.[3] These lie at the base of the spine; over the solar

[1] Sometimes referred to in the West as the etheric body. The Indian term is *linga-deha* or *linga-śarīra*.
[2] *Some Unrecognized Factors in Medicine* (Theosophical Research Centre London), p. 15.
[3] The function of the subtle bodies and their centres or etheric organs is both psychological and physiological. For the purposes of the Yoga only the psychological aspect is treated here, but those interested

plexus; the spleen and heart; in front of the throat; between the eyebrows and over the top of the head.

The specialized action of each centre is defined by Sri Aurobindo as follows: the base of spine (*mūlādhāra*) governs the physical down to the subconscient.[1] The abdominal centre (*svādhiṣṭhāna*) governs the small sense-movements. The navel centre (*maṇipura*) governs the larger desire-movements. The heart centre (*hṛtpadma* or *anāhata*) governs the emotional being. The throat centre (*viśuddha*) governs the expressive and externalizing mind. The centre between the eyebrows (*ājñacakra*) governs the dynamic will, vision, mental formation; the thousand-petalled lotus (*sahasradala*), above the head, commands the higher thinking mind, houses the still higher illumined mind, and at the highest opens to the intuition, through which the Overmind can have communication or immediate contact with the rest.

The mental and vital sheaths or bodies are supported inwardly by the soul. They are also linked with vital and mental planes above the material universe.

In the operation of the mental and vital being of the individual, Sri Aurobindo distinguishes between the surface action, as it is involved in the egotistical expression of mind, life and body, and the true nature of their function. Thus "the surface vital (being) is narrow, ignorant,

in the physiological side may find it described in the above-mentioned book. (See also *Country Life*: "Telepathy: a Suggestion" (June 23, 1950) and "The Problem of Human Radiations" (April 13, 1951) by O. Bagnall).

[1] "In our Yoga we mean by the subconscient that quite submerged part of our being in which there is no wakingly conscious and coherent thought, will or feeling or organized reaction, but which yet receives obscurely the impressions of all things and stores them up in itself and from it too all sorts of stimuli, of persistent habitual movements, crudely repeated or disguised in strange forms, can surge up into dreams or into the waking nature. In the subconscient there is an obscure mind full of obstinate samskaras formed by our past, an obscure vital full of the seeds of habitual desires, sensations, and nervous reactions, a most obscure material which governs much that has to do with the conditions of the body." (*Lights on Yoga*, pp. 11-12.)

limited, full of obscure desires, passions, cravings, revolts, pleasures and pains, transient joys and griefs, exultations and depression. The true vital being, on the contrary, is wide, vast, calm, strong, without limitations, firm and immovable, capable of all power, all knowledge, all Ananda. It is moreover without ego, for it knows itself to be a projection and instrument of the Divine. . . . In the same way there is, too, a true mental being, a true physical being. When these are manifest, then you are aware of a double existence in you: that behind is always calm and strong, that on the surface alone is troubled and obscure."[1] He goes on to say that though the action of the mind and vital being are mixed up on the surface of consciousness, they are quite separate forces in themselves and must be carefully distinguished.

The mental being connotes specially that part of the nature which has to do with "cognition and intelligence, with ideas, with mental or thought perceptions, the re-action of thought to things, with the truly mental move-ments and formations, mental vision and will, etc., that are part of . . . intelligence".

The vital being, on the other hand, "is the life nature made up of desires, sensations, feelings, passions, energies of action, will of desire, reactions of the desire soul in man and of all that play of possessive and other related in-stincts, anger, fear, greed, lust, etc., that belong to this field of the nature".[2] The division or conflict between the

---

[1] *Lights on Yoga*, p. 13.
[2] Ibid., pp. 14-15.
"There are four parts of the vital being—first, the mental vital which gives a mental expression by thought, speech or otherwise to the emo-tions, desires, passions, sensations and other movements of the vital being; the emotional vital which is the seat of various feelings such as love, joy, sorrow, hatred, and the rest; the central vital which is the seat of the stronger vital longings and reactions, e.g. ambition, pride, fear, love of fame, attractions and repulsions, desires and passions of various kinds and the field of many vital energies; last, the lower vital which is occupied with small desires and feelings, such as make the greater

mental and vital principles, he adds, is the cause of most of the more acute difficulties in the practice of the Yoga, for while one part of the nature may accept the ideal placed before it, the other may stubbornly refuse to surrender.

It is perhaps a risk to try and equate these precise psychological terms with the vague distinctions of Western psychology, but in order to try and clarify for the reader the difference between the true mental and vital being and their surface action when it is an expression of the ego, it may be suggested that there is a rough analogy here to Jung's concept of the 'shadow'.

The substitution of the true mental and vital being for the action of the lower, and the opening of the *chakras* or subtle centres to higher forces of consciousness, is a central part of the process of Integral Yoga, and more will be said of this later. It will suffice here to add that in the opening of the centres Sri Aurobindo's method differs from those Yogas which, like the Tantric, detail a specific discipline and purification, the opening accomplishing itself naturally as a result of the processes of the Yoga.

Described in this bald and cataloguing manner, the psychology of the individual may appear difficult and complicated. In fact, the various planes and levels of consciousness and organization of the being can only be realized effectively by deepening experience. It would seem, to such an extending knowledge of spiritual experience, that these psychological distinctions take on an ever-increasing significance and subtlety, both in their individual and cosmic aspects, far more wonderful and

part of daily life, e.g. food desire, sexual desire, small likings, dislikings, vanity, quarrels, love of praise, anger at blame, little wishes of all kinds —and a numberless host of other things. Their respective seats are (i) the region from the throat to the heart, (ii) the heart (it is a double centre, belonging in front to the emotional and vital and behind to the psychic [being]), (iii) from the heart to the navel, (iv) below the navel. (*Letters*, Vol.I, p. 170.)

complex than we can possibly imagine while we remain involved in the outward, surface action of our natures.

Before leaving this brief outline of the psychology on which Integral Yoga is based, it would be well to make clear that Sri Aurobindo's teaching does not in any way aim at the 'annihilation' of personality, so often imputed (usually ignorantly) to Eastern mysticism. It aims at the transformation of personality into the image of an original perfection already inherent in the divine nature of man: for behind true personality stands the Divine Person.

The Supreme Being contains "an apparent vast Impersonal"[1] which may be characterized in the contemplative act by a sense of ineffable silence and immobility, but this is only one aspect of His reality. The Divine is also the essence and source of all pure personality, therefore an Infinite Person, "a Master of our works, a Friend and Lover of our soul, an intimate Spirit of our life".[2] This loving relation of the Supreme Person with the soul is exemplified in the relationship between the divine Krishna and Arjuna in the *Gita*. "Thou art exceedingly beloved of Me," Krishna tells Arjuna, "therefore I will say what is for thy weal. . . . To Me shalt thou come. I make thee a truthful promise; thou art dear to me."[3] Again, the *Swetaswatara Upanishad* speaks of the joy of the soul when it is in union "with that other self and greatness of it which is the Lord".

But, Sri Aurobindo warns, we must not confuse Person with our experience of ego. "Nothing is more difficult for us than to get rid of egoism while yet we admit personality," he writes in *The Synthesis of Yoga*.[4] And speaking of man's true relation to God, he says that man is "a centre only—a centre of differentiation of the one personal con-

[1] *Essays on the Gita* (Second Series), p. 381.
[2] Ibid., p. 369.
[3] *Bhagavad Gita* 18, vv. 64-5.
[4] *The Synthesis of Yoga*, p. 246.

sciousness . . . his personality reflects in a wave of persistent individuality the one universal Person, the Transcendent, the Eternal". But while man remains tied to his lower nature, he adds, "it is always a broken and distorted reflection".[1] Therefore the aim of Integral Yoga is to strip from the individual all the flawed conditions which corrupt the divine image and in so doing to liberate the true Person, who is alone capable of receiving that reflection in all its completeness, purity and perfection.

[1] *The Synthesis of Yoga*, p. 173.

CHAPTER III

THE TRIPLE ASCENT

The object of the Yoga is to enter into and be possessed
by the Divine Presence and Consciousness, to love the
Divine for the Divine's sake alone, to be turned in our
nature into the nature of the Divine, and in our will and
works and life to be the instrument of the Divine.
Letters, Vol. II, p. 3.

And this great thing, to rise from the human into the
Divine nature, we can only do by an effort of Godward
knowledge, will and adoration. . . .
Perfection cannot come without self-knowledge and
God-knowledge. . . . The soul's salvation cannot come without the soul's perfection, without its growing into the
divine nature. . . . Divine works are effective for salvation
because they lead us towards this perfection and to a
knowledge of self and nature and God by a growing unity
with the inner Master of our existence. Divine love is
effective because by it we grow into the likeness of the sole
and supreme object of our adoration and call down the
answering love of the Highest to flood us with the light of
his knowledge and the uplifting power and purity of his
eternal spirit.
Essays on the Gita (Second Series), pp. 213–14.

DESCRIBED briefly, the aim of Integral Yoga might be
summed up as the transformation of the mental into the
spiritual being: but the word 'transformation', which we
have used so far in a general way, to indicate the change
to be effected by the Yoga, has a very precise definition
for Sri Aurobindo.

"I use transformation in a special sense" (he says), "a
change of consciousness *radical and complete* and of a

62

certain specific kind. . . . A partial realization, something mixed and inconclusive, does not meet the demand I make on life and Yoga."[1] It is, in brief, an *integral*[2] transformation, requiring that every level of the individual consciousness should be purified and illumined, mental, vital and physical, the outer as well as the inner consciousness. For, he points out, it is possible to achieve liberation, to attain realization, without either the vital or physical consciousness changing at all, and this indeed has been achieved by contemplatives, working under various mystical disciplines, since time began.

But as we have seen, Integral Yoga is not concerned simply with individual liberation. It aims, through a descent of the higher powers of consciousness into the entire being, at a definitive change in the earth consciousness and takes "fulfilment of the life and body for its object," and of the whole nexus of mind, life and body for the field of the divine action in time. This descent Sri Aurobindo describes as the main key of the spiritual transformation and nothing can be done without it. He therefore characterizes the movement of the Yoga as one of ascent and descent, and its specific action as synthetic —a taking up of the whole being into the divine consciousness.

But he insists that this descent is not to be confused with realization. "Realization by itself does not necessarily transform the being as a whole; it may bring only an opening or heightening or widening of consciousness at the top,"[3] and this, though it may affect the psychic nature, leaves the natural or physical consciousness unchanged.

He observes that he has seen many cases of this

[1] *Letters*, Vol. I, p. 23. My italics.
[2] "Integral Yoga, that is, a turning of the being in all its parts to the Divine." (*Letters*, Vol. II, p. 4.)
[3] *Letters*, Vol. I, p. 23.

happen, and goes on to say: "There must be a descent of the light not merely into the mind or part of it but into all the being down to the physical and below before a real transformation can take place. A light in the mind may spiritualize or otherwise change the mind or part of it in one way or another, but it need not change the vital nature; a light in the vital (being) may purify and enlarge the vital movements or else silence and immobilize the vital being, but leave the body and the physical consciousness as it was, or even leave it inert or shake its balance. And the descent of Light is not enough, it must be the descent of the whole higher consciousness, its Peace, Power, Knowledge, Love, Ananda[1] . . . Psychicization (i.e. the control of the being by the soul) is not enough, it is only a beginning; spiritualization and the descent of the higher consciousness is not enough, it is only a middle term; the ultimate achievement needs the action of the Supramental Consciousness and Force. Something less than that may very well be considered enough by the individual, but it is not enough for the earth-consciousness to take the definitive stride forward it must take at one time or another."[2]

This final consideration alone might be thought sufficient to establish the necessity of these exacting demands, but there is another, repeatedly stressed by Sri Aurobindo. The descent of the Divine Force into a mind and vital being not prepared for it may lead to serious disturbance and even danger. Therefore he insists over and over again on purification and sanctification as the "great necessities of sadhana".[3] "Those who have experiences before purification," he warns a disciple, "run a great risk"; and again: "To try to bring down occult powers into an unpurified mind, heart and body—well,

---

[1] The Sanskrit term *ananda* means spiritual delight, bliss, ecstasy.
[2] *Letters*, Vol. I, pp. 24-5.
[3] *Sadhana*: yogic practice.

you can do it if you want to dance on the edge of a precipice."[1]

Integral Yoga, then, requires of those who practise it a total transformation and indicates as its central object in obtaining this goal an ascent of the individual consciousness towards the Divine, and a descent of the Divine Consciousness into the individual. Because it is synthetic in character, it requires that the surrender of the heart should bring to the Divine the sacrifice[2] of love; the surrender of the mind, the sacrifice of knowledge and will; the surrender of the vital being, the sacrifice of works. These three great offerings are the main support of the Yoga and form the way of a triple ascent.

The *Karma Yoga* of the *Bhagavad Gita*, on which Integral Yoga is based, calls this ascent the union of knowledge, works, and love, and in it, Sri Aurobindo tells us, the full active life of man is perfectly reconciled with the inner life in the highest self and spirit.[3]

It is therefore necessary, before approaching what might be called the minutiae of the Yoga—the actual *sadhana* or practice—to understand Sri Aurobindo's interpretation of this sovereign way to God of the *karmayogin*, expounded with such infinite beauty and subtlety in the *Gita*, since it is the framework into which the spiritual practice of Integral Yoga is built.

---

[1] *Letters*, Vol. II, p. 331.

[2] Sacrifice in its spiritual sense, meaning *to make sacred* or sanctify.

[3] The pattern of this way of grace with its triune requirement of knowledge, devotion and will is also apparent in the Fourth Gospel. Jesus clearly enunciated it as the great Word which lay at the core of His spiritual way in His reply to the Pharisee lawyer, when he tempted Him: "Thou shalt love the Lord thy God with all thy heart, and with all thy soul, and with all thy mind." St. Matthew, Ch. xxii, v. 37.

CHAPTER IV

KNOWLEDGE, WORKS AND LOVE:

THE WAY OF THE KARMAYOGIN

> To see nothing but the Divine, to be at every moment in union with him, to love him in all creatures and have the delight of him in all things is the whole condition of his (the spiritual man's) existence. His God-vision does not divorce him from life, nor does he miss any of the fulness of life; for God himself becomes the spontaneous bringer to him of every good. . . . The joy of heaven and the joy of earth are only a small shadow of his possessions; for as he grows into the Divine, the Divine too flows out upon him with all the light, power and joy of an infinite existence.
>
> *Essays on the Gita* (Second Series), p. 93.

> This is the Gita's teaching of divine love and devotion, in which knowledge, works and the heart's longing become one in a supreme unification, a merging of all their divergences, an intertwining of all their threads. . . .
>
> *Essays on the Gita* (Second Series), p. 99.

> This is not a Yoga of Bhakti (devotion) alone, it is or at least it claims to be an integral Yoga, that is, a turning of the being in all its parts to the Divine. . . . It is not only the heart that has to turn to the Divine and change, but the mind also—so knowledge is necessary and the will and power of action and creation also—so works too are necessary.
>
> *Letters*, Vol. II, p. 4.

THE spiritual way of the *Gita* is one of affirmation. It does not place an exclusive emphasis on action or contemplation, neither does it give pre-eminence to works, nor to a quietistic withdrawal from action, as the royal way to God. Negative passivity, the renunciation of life and works, is admitted, "but only with a minor, permissive sanction",[1] Sri Aurobindo observes. It is the driest and most difficult way to God; the way of "the razor's edge".

Against intolerant asceticism or pride of knowledge it sets its face firmly, as also against a "passive relationless identity (which) excludes love and action".[2] A diminution of works is not indispensable; it is not even advisable; it may be a dangerous example. This idea is elaborated by Sri Aurobindo in *The Life Divine* also, where he urges that the passive and dynamic aspects, being part of the Divine Being, must also represent the perfect human pattern. Not cessation from action, but renunciation from desire is the guiding principle of the *Gita*. The Integral Way lies in the perfect synthesis of knowledge, works and love. The pattern of its following is in the manner in which Arjuna accepts the truth "with the adoration of his heart, the submission of his will and the understanding of his intelligence".[3]

This knowledge is not mental cognizance, but evolution into a higher spiritual consciousness, a knowledge of heart and spirit. Salvation, which is dependent on perfection, cannot come without self-knowledge and only ascent into a higher principle of consciousness can bring that self-knowledge and God-knowledge.[4]

To withdraw the soul from outward concentration in the ego to inward union with God is the way of liberation. This turning inward to seek God is the first condition on which the *Gita's* *sadhana* is built. It is necessary, therefore, to remember the exact distinctions we gave to Self, soul and ego-personality in Chapter II if we wish to follow

[1] *Essays on the Gita* (Second Series), p. 105.
[2] Ibid., p. 109.
[3] Ibid., p. 127.
[4] "Knowledge in this sense is an awakening to identity", that is, with the Divine Truth-Consciousness. *Essays on the Gita* (Second Series), p. 84.

the psychological directions of the *Gita's* teaching. It is the extinction of the ego with its divided consciousness and avid desires which the mysticism of the *Gita* enjoins, and the withdrawal of the soul into the primordial purity and unity of God, whose kingdom is within.

The first step, then, is the development of the *sattwic*[1] qualities of goodness, humility, chastity, compassion, and the attainment of inner quietness and impersonality. The divisions and ignorance of the ego, together with sin—the revolt of the *rajasic* propensities against the mastery of the spirit—must all be overcome.

But ethical action to the *Gita* is only a means of self-purification. Man can never attain to the highest by virtue alone, though by its practice he can develop a first capacity for attainment. When the aspirant has achieved this equanimity and perfect inner immobility, he must next offer his action to God as a sacrifice. The idea of himself as the author of the action will still persist, but the fruits will be offered to God. He will no longer seize them personally as his own. Failure and success, praise or blame will not disturb his impersonal calm. All will be offered up to the Lord of the Sacrifice.

Thirdly he will act, but surrender all notion of himself as the doer, acting in the consciousness that it is the energy-force (or power of manifestation) of God which is the sole doer. He will act in the knowledge of this force as God's supreme power and in a renunciation, a surrender, of all actions to their Source, seeing himself only as a channel for their effectuation in the world.

All sense of action as being individual will cease. United then with God in knowledge and in works, in mind

---

[1] The action of Nature subjects the soul, while it is still attached to the Ignorance, to three modes or *Gunas*, which are her qualities, *sattwa*, *rajas*, and *tamas*. Psychologically these can be defined roughly as contemplative mental type (*sattwic*), active type (*rajasic*) and ignorant, inert type (*tamasic*). In Nature Sri Aurobindo defines them as equilibrium, kinesis, inertia.

and will, he will act, not from egoistic choice, but from the Truth-Consciousness of the Divine and Eternal Being which will possess him.

There is yet a further step the disciple must take. He must know God as "the One who eternally becomes the Many, the Many who in their apparent division are still eternally one".[1] He must know that there is no dichotomy of being itself, but "a multiplicity of status of the one Being"[2] in all his relations of difference.

This integral knowledge comes only by love: "a highest bhakti[3]. . . that is calm and deep and luminous with widest knowledge".[4] This profound love of the soul, "its heart's knowledge", is the core of the integral beatitude, "when the heart's fathomless vision completes the mind's absolute experience".[5]

When man has once seen this vision of his true nature and of God as the Supreme Being, Creator of the universe and all beings, "his whole life aspiration becomes a surpassing love and fathomless adoration of the Divine".[6]

Thus, says Krishna, the divine Teacher, this supreme vision "cannot be won by Veda or austerities or gifts or sacrifice; it can be seen, known, entered into only by that bhakti which regards, adores and loves Me in all things".[7]

Love is the crown of works and the crown of knowledge. Perfect love is the key to perfect knowledge. Its supreme seal on life is reflected by man living in the world for God.

The teaching of the *Gita*—and likewise of Integral Yoga—points then to the perfection of the being through an offering of the whole existence in which heart, mind and will are fully integrated. Through it we are bidden to

[1] *Essays on the Gita* (Second Series), p. 363.
[2] *The Life Divine*, Vol. II (1), p. 237.
[3] *Bhakti*: devotion.
[4] *Essays on the Gita* (Second Series), p. 363.
[5] Ibid.
[6] Ibid., p. 87.
[7] *Bhagavad Gita*: Lesson XI, vv. 53-4.

put on the true spiritual nature; the nature of those who live, move and have their being *consciously* in God, and to lose the life of the ego. In this redeemed life the Elect are *all* those, even the most hopeless and sinful, who can make that initial act of self-surrender. "If," says Krishna, "even a man of very evil conduct turns to Me with a sole and entire love . . . (he will) obtain eternal peace."[1]

On the subject of love the psychological scrutiny of the *Gita* is, however, very piercing. There are many subtle corruptions of the egoistic nature—even of the sattwic, the highest ethical nature—which must be watched over.

The disciple must not fall into the self-centredness which seeks an egoistic seclusion from the trouble of participation in the world-action. Neither must he fall into any error of partial love for God. And partial love means for the *Gita* that love which turns to God for succour or deliverance in suffering; which seeks Him for His gifts, or for aid and protection; or which, still ignorant, turns to Him for knowledge and illumination. So long as the disciple is limited to these forms there may persist even in the highest and noblest endeavour a working of the three *gunas*.

In brief, God must be loved and adored for Himself. Here the object of the *Gita's* constant emphasis on knowledge is made clear. Though love brings the supreme knowledge (truth-consciousness), love without knowledge is a snare.

This may seem a paradox. It means simply that the highest *bhakti* cannot come unless it is based upon a real discernment of the nature of God, man and the cosmos. A man cannot act in truth unless the ground of his action is a perfect knowledge. The fruit of the spiritual life "is according to the knowledge, the faith and the work and cannot exceed their limitations".[2]

[1] *Bhagavad Gita*: Lesson IX, vv. 29-30.
[2] *Essays on the Gita* (Second Series), p. 94.

In this process the *Gita* stresses the need for each individual to find and follow the unique inner law—*swadharma*—of his own being, which in turn possesses its own law of progress. Even if it is defective it is better than the well-performed rule of another's nature. This inward law is the being's natural way of evolution and to follow any other is dangerous.

In the forward adventure of faith a man's guiding light will be "his will to believe, to live what he thinks or sees to be the truth of himself and of existence",[1] for this rises from a divine formulation in him which he must develop. It is an inner guidance to act and think the truth; not obedience to a compulsive standard of belief thrust upon him by church or state, but freedom to hear and follow the intimate direction of God in his own heart.

If he is to hear that inner voice clearly and to learn to distinguish it from the ego, which will seek slyly to simulate it, he must take up the work of the Yoga with the utmost sincerity and purity of intention of which he is capable.

---

[1] *Essays on the Gita*, p. 289.

PART II

The Practice of the Yoga

CHAPTER I

SURRENDER

To give oneself is the secret of sadhana.
Letters, Vol. I, p. 269.
For surrender, everyone has his own first way of
approach towards it. . . . Complete and total surrender is
not so easy as some seem to imagine. There are always
many and large reservations; even if one is not conscious of
them, they are there. Complete surrender can best come by
a complete love and bhakti. Bhakti, on the other hand, can
begin without surrender, but it naturally leads, as it forms
itself, to surrender.   *Letters*, Vol. II, p. 339.
It is only when the surrender is complete that the full
flood of the sadhana is possible.   *Letters*, Vol. II, p. 5.
It is said in the 'Sanatsujatiya' that four things are
needed for perfection . . . the teaching of the path, zeal in
following it, the Master and time.
The Yoga and its Objects, p. 47.
At the beginning one should not ask for any other fruit
or result than . . . internal growth or change.
Bases of Yoga, p. 33.
Eliminate egoism in all its forms; eliminate it from
every movement of your consciousness.
Bases of Yoga, p. 44.

FOLLOWING the outlines of the *Gita's* Yoga, Sri Aurobindo defines the spiritual movement towards Divine
realization as divided into three processes.
Firstly, there must be made by the aspirant an act of
self-consecration to the Divine (*samarpaṇa*). Secondly, he
must learn by detachment and self-knowledge to see that
it is God who works in him, and to renounce all idea of

75

possessing a separate independence. And thirdly, he must perceive all things and happenings as God. In love he will aim at purification of the heart and intellect; in action, at self-surrender in all things and at every moment to God; and in knowledge at realization of the One within, and beyond all manifested existence.

In effect, these three movements may often develop together, or in a different order, depending on the nature of the aspirant, the *bhakta* going more speedily along the road of the heart (*bhakta yoga*) and the thinker more easily along the road of knowledge (*jnana yoga*).

They represent the wide sweeps of the ascent, the great contours that distinguish the Holy Mountain, to which the aspirant can lift his eyes in order to acquaint himself with the terrain of his heavenly adventure, knowing that every step forward on the ascent will have to be carefully planned and often laboriously and painstakingly cut out in the many precipice faces that await him.

Get the broad outlines of the campaign in your head first, Sri Aurobindo would seem to advise, then settle down patiently to working out every stage of the movement, detail by detail as the Divine directs you. Remember that though the general lines are common to all, each nature is unique and has its own method of following the way. The Divine Master will treat each one with ineffable tact, working to transform each nature by the way of its own inner law, which is also the personal formulation of His delight in it, through which He experiences differentiation in His divine play.

Begin, he says, by making an act of surrender and dedication. "Put yourself with all your heart and strength into God's hands. Make no conditions, ask for nothing, not even for perfection in the Yoga, for nothing at all except that in you and through you His will may be directly performed."[1]

[1] *The Yoga and Its Objects*, p. 9.

In order to make this surrender complete, nothing must be reserved. There must be no self-will in demanding or desiring this or that, no egotistical clinging to preconceived ideas about how the Yoga should go. Indeed, the core of the surrender is precisely a yielding up of this determination, which forms such a tough centre in each one of us, to see things and to act in the half-light of our own theories and preconceptions.

The tenacity and subtlety with which each individual's particular forms of egotism disguise themselves against detection makes a total surrender at the beginning of the *sadhana* impossible to most natures. "A complete surrender means to cut the knot of the ego in each part of the being and offer it, free and whole, to the Divine. The mind, the vital (being), the physical consciousness (and even each part of these in all its movements) have one after the other to surrender separately, to give up their own way and to accept the way of the Divine."[1]

Such a surrender is not possible at the beginning, save for a few; nevertheless, so important is the working out of this movement that it is worth studying exhaustively. Were it possible to achieve it perfectly, Sri Aurobindo observes, the necessity for a special discipline in the Yoga would disappear, and he emphasizes its vital rôle in the *sadhana* by saying that to those who can make the full surrender from the beginning the path is utterly swift and easy.

For the average individual the act of surrender must be progressive, something he learns to deepen, widen and heighten as he detects the resistances in his own nature and comes to feel the Divine Presence more closely and with it a more intense need of self-giving.

In this early stage Sri Aurobindo suggests that the best thing to do is "to make from the beginning a central resolve and self-dedication and to implement it in what-

[1] *Bases of Yoga*, p. 32.

ever way one finds open, at each step, taking advantage of each occasion that offers itself to make the self-giving complete. A surrender in one direction makes others easier, more inevitable; but it does not of itself cut or loosen the other knots, and especially those which are very intimately bound up with the present personality, and its most cherished formations may often present great difficulties, even after the central will has been fixed and the first seals put on its resolve in practice."[1]

He calls this inner and outer surrender "the central process of the Yoga", its "first principle", and repeats that it is a putting of oneself "in the hands of the Divine rather than relying on one's own efforts alone and this implies one's putting one's trust and confidence in the Divine and a progressive selfgiving".[2] This trust and confidence is "the core of the inner surrender".[3] It is based on the heart, on a self-offering of love to God. The more one gives oneself, he says, the more the power to receive will grow; but in order to do this, all demand, impatience, rebelliousness, depression and discouragement at setbacks, must be put aside.

He does not conceal the difficulties. "Because it is difficult," he writes, "it has to be done steadily and patiently till the work is complete,"[4] and he insists again and again that it is the basic principle of the *sadhana* without which its fulfilment is impossible.

Patience, faith, steadfastness and an intense, quiet and hopeful aspiration are the qualities best calculated to sustain each one. All must be given up or rejected that conflicts with the spirit or necessity of the *sadhana*. There must be a constant endeavour to obey the guidance of the Divine, whether through the direction of the human

[1] *Bases of Yoga*, p. 32.
[2] *Letters*, Vol. I, p. 77.
[3] Ibid., p. 78.
[4] Ibid., Vol. IV, p. 139.

Teacher, through the intimations given by the soul, or by the Divine Himself.

These three instruments of Divine guidance concern rather different stages in the Yoga and we will return to them again later. It is sufficient to emphasize here that the taking up directly of the *sadhana* by the Divine, which should spring centrally from the methods of this Yoga, only becomes possible through the gradual perfecting of the initial act of surrender.

Though it may not be easy to make at first anything but a partial self-offering, the fuller it becomes, so the Divine help and guidance increase accordingly. Such a self-giving releases the being from the exclusive concentration and pursuit of its own viewpoint, interests and desires, natural to the ego, and opens it to the operation of the Divine Force.

The obstacles, difficulties and dangers that lie in the way of this spiritual movement are those characteristic, in some shape, of every stage in the development of the Yoga so long as any trace of egotism remains.

While the right attitude is growing, wrong movements from the vital and mental being may continually disturb, but if the will and aspiration are kept firm, the right attitude will gradually establish itself. "The rest," Sri Aurobindo observes, "is a matter of obedience to the guidance when it makes itself manifest, not allowing one's mental and vital movements to interfere."[1]

In a sense, all the broad, basic movements of the Yoga overlap one another and the power to stand apart from the *adhara*[2]—to learn to distinguish the different parts of one's being without identifying oneself with their outward action—which first makes possible the direct

---

[1] *Letters*, Vol. I, pp. 78-9.
[2] *Adhara*: "Vessel, receptacle—the system of mind, life and body considered as a receptacle of the spiritual consciousness and force." (*More Lights on Yoga*, p. 135.)

guidance of the Divine, is also indispensable in this early stage.

Each individual finds different resistances in his nature. Some find the most stubborn obstacles in surrendering the mind, others in surrendering the vital being. Typical difficulties associated with the first are doubt, a universal malaise in this age in nearly every aspirant, Eastern or Western, Sri Aurobino remarks: also intellectual fault-finding with the teaching; the wish to follow one's own ideas; opinionation, arrogance and so on.

Difficulties associated with the emotional, or vital, nature usually prove the most persistent and hard to eradicate, particularly those of the lower vital being, which, through the chakra at the base of the spine (*muladhara*), is linked with the powerful life-force and its action in animal sex-energy.

Temper, irritation, impatience, restlessness are all obvious faults connected with wrong vital movements, as are greed, desire, vanity and ambition. With patience it is possible to distinguish which subtle centres are responding to particular stimuli. For instance, fear is often felt as an unpleasant turning over of the stomach, due to a rapid reversal in the movement of the solar plexus chakra (*manipura*); while nervousness or embarrassment frequently produce a stricture of the throat, caused by the throat chakra (*visuddha*) suddenly tightening.

In creative work or meditation, the forehead (*ajna*) and overhead (*sahasradala*)[1] chakras can sometimes be felt acting, but these sensations are very much more delicate and subtle.[2] It is not enough, we are told, to have a general consciousness of ignorance and obscurity; it must be

---

[1] The *sahasradala* chakra "is sometimes called the void centre, *sunya*, either because it is not in the body, but in the apparent void above, or because rising above the head one enters first into the silence of the self or spiritual being". (*More Lights on Yoga*, p. 36.)
[2] The symbol of the opening of the centres to the Light is the lotus. (*Letters*, Vol. IV, p. 333.)

known in its details and actual working before wrong movements can be rejected.

The dangers that beset the path before the surrender is complete are described in detail by Sri Aurobindo. Because it is necessary in the early stages, before the Divine Presence takes up the *sadhana* itself, to make a strong personal effort, great vigilance must be used in not placing too much reliance on this effort. It must be "an effort in which there is the spirit of surrender, calling in the Force to support the will and effort and undisturbed by success or failure".[1]

Few are strong enough to overcome the forces of the lower nature by their own will. Indeed, unaided effort can effect nothing but disaster, for no one may cross from ignorance to truth save by grace. While a sincere, steadfast and humble personal endeavour is required in the early stages of the *sadhana*, the aim must always be that this effort should gradually be taken up by the Divine Force; until then it must be made "with an increasing reality of surrender",[2] calling in and trusting to the Divine Grace at every step, by aspiration, concentration or prayer.

Too great a reliance on personal effort is the danger of the *rajoguna*, into which the active type of individual may most readily fall. It may lead to pride; to the belief that the disciple is a great *sadhaka* (i.e. one who practises the discipline of Yoga), a great instrument in God's hands, and to the attachment to the work as God's work—something he has been missioned to carry out, and other forms of self-assertive egoism.

Likewise, too early an abandonment of individual effort, in the belief that the Divine has taken up the work, may lead to the danger of the *tamoguna*, in which inertia and indolence and inactivity are mistaken for peace: or

[1] *Letters*, Vol. IV, p. 130.
[2] Ibid., Vol. II, p. 5.

another error of the *tamoguna* in which the soul identifies itself with the inertia in the being and adopts an attitude of helplessness and impotence, imagining that God will not be able to deal with its incapacities.

Then there are the subtle deceptions of the *sattva guna* to which the highest ethical, naturally contemplative type may fall a prey. Here the aspirant may become attached to some particular aspect of the Yoga, to joy or delight or the possession of a special power: to the desire for liberation or contact with God.

All these illusions are in some way present in each one of us. All suffer in the early stages from what Sri Aurobindo describes as "the haunting idea of sin and virtue". Remember, he adds, "that since you have put yourself in God's hands, He will work out the impurities and you have only to be careful, as you cannot be attached either to sin or virtue. For He has repeatedly given the assurance of safety. He says in the *Gita*, 'He who is devoted to Me cannot perish.'[1]"

There is another danger before the surrender is complete. This is the danger of being two people, of being in two minds, and it persists wherever there is an equivocality in the dedication. For instance, the mind may turn itself towards God, while a sanction still exists secretly for the vital nature to make its demands and fulfil its desires.

Again, there may be a temptation to give one part of the life to the Divine, while reserving the rest of it for the old ways and pursuits, a course fatal to success in the Yoga and a special danger for those who choose to practise it in the world without the support of the discipline imposed on a community.

Only vigilance can detect these things and single-mindedness make their occurrence impossible. Therefore, says Sri Aurobindo, in Yoga there is one indispensable condition—sincerity.

[1] *The Yoga and Its Objects*, p. 31.

For the rest, he advises, the right attitude for the beginner to take is this: "I want the Divine and nothing else. I want to give myself entirely to him and since my soul wants that, it cannot be but that I shall meet and realize him. I ask nothing but that and his action secret or open, veiled or manifest. I do not insist on my own time and way. Let him do all in his own time and way; I shall believe in him, accept his will, aspire steadily for his light and presence and joy, go through all difficulties and delays, relying on him and never giving up. Let my mind be quiet and turn to him alone and let him open it to his light; let my vital (being) be quiet and turn to him alone and let him open it to his calm and joy. All for him and myself for him. Whatever happens I will keep to this aspiration and self-giving and go on in perfect reliance that it will be done."[1]

Above all, he says, be patient. This is the most difficult and complex Yoga and it can only be done by stages; time is needed, particularly at the beginning, and by time he means, not days or weeks or even months, but years. To a discouraged disciple he once wrote: "Eight years is a very short time for transformation. Most people spend as much as that or more to get conscious of their defects and acquire the serious will to change—and after that it takes a long time to get the will turned into full and final accomplishment."[2]

All the great vocations of man require a lifetime of tireless endeavour for their perfection. What is demanded of the great soldier, poet, musician, or scientist is demanded in increased measure of the mystic.

[1] *Letters*, Vol. I, p. 78.
[2] Ibid., Vol. IV, p. 142.

CHAPTER II

THE QUIET MIND

Remember first that an inner quietude, caused by the purification of the restless mind and vital, is the first condition of a secure sadhana.   *Bases of Yoga*, pp. 21-22.

Aspire especially for quietness, peace, a calm faith, an increasing steady wideness, for more and more knowledge, for a deep and intense but quiet devotion.
Ibid., p. 16.

The path of Yoga is always beset with inner and outer difficulties and the sadhaka must develop a quiet, firm and solid strength to meet them.
Ibid., p. 17.

Not only a truer knowledge, but a greater power comes to one in the quietude and silence of a mind that, instead of bubbling on the surface, can go to its own depths and listen.   *Letters*, Vol. II, p. 152.

Peace and calmness are the first thing, and with it the wideness—in the peace you can bear whatever love or Ananda comes, whatever strength comes or whatever knowledge.   *More Lights on Yoga*, p. 95.

THE first and best foundation on which to start the work of Integral Yoga is a quiet mind. The qualities of peace, purity and calm are the basic necessities without which nothing else can safely be built. The true consciousness, Sri Aurobindo maintains, can only be created in a silent mind, for where there is no peace or quietness, experiences, when they come, cannot be permanent. Worse still, occurring in an unpurified and disturbed consciousness, they will be full of disorder and mixture and lead the aspirant into confusion.

84

Equability can only result from inner quietness, and without equability there can be no standing back from the external nature and no power to remain unshaken or undisturbed in the midst of adverse conditions. "When the mind is quiet and at peace the Force can work more easily,"[1] he writes; but when the mind is continually invaded by troubling thoughts, wrong feelings, confusion of ideas, unhappy movements, the nature becomes clouded and these conditions make it difficult for the Force to act undisturbed.

The surface mind is always at the mercy of the shocks and blows of life. To go increasingly and more deeply within and to seek there the calm of the inner being is to cease to be involved in the fret of this surface consciousness, for "it is only from that inner state that one can be stronger than life and its disturbing forces and hope to conquer".[2]

To be detached from the turmoil of surface mental activity and from the movements of the vital being; to be able to discriminate between the experiences of the inner self and the play of the outer nature, is an indispensable step in the Yoga and none of this can be done, or kept constant, without being calm, steady, fixed in spirit.

Calm, he says, is the very nature of the Supreme Being and the positive foundation of the divine consciousness, and whatever else is aspired for and gained, this must be kept. If the divine powers of knowledge, power and bliss descend and do not find this foundation they are unable to remain and have to withdraw.

The consciousness of peace in mind, life and body and surrounding the individual everywhere is the sure sign of the Divine's presence, and once possessed, all the rest will begin to come. But this all-pervading consciousness of

[1] *Bases of Yoga*, p. 3.
[2] Ibid., p. 17.

peace is not to be attained all at once or even very easily. The safest and most favourable approach is to begin by quietening the mind; therefore, Sri Aurobindo urges, make the attainment of this "the first thing" in the *sadhana*.

As the two great agents of Yoga are a "pressure of understanding and will in the mind"[1] and an intense urge of devotion towards God in the heart, so is its basis this purity and peace which springs from the quiet mind and finally possesses the whole individual and all his activities.[2]

Sri Aurobindo defines a quiet mind as one "that does not involve itself in its thoughts or get run away with by them; it stands back, detaches itself, lets them pass without identifying itself, without making them its own. It becomes the witness mind watching the thoughts when necessary but able to turn away from them and receive from within and from above."[3] Quietness does not mean that there will be no thoughts or mental movements at all, neither is it the same thing as silence, which concerns a more advanced stage of the Yoga. Silence is always good, but it is not indispensable at the beginning.

Quietness means "a mind free from disturbance and trouble, steady, light and glad so as to be open to the Force that will change the nature".[4] It is characterized by this sense of standing apart and in detachment becoming conscious of the inner being or soul as separate from the action of the ordinary nature.

"If thoughts or activities take place in the quiet mind," Sri Aurobindo writes, "they do not rise at all out of the mind, but they come from outside and cross the mind as a flight of birds crosses the sky in a windless air. It passes,

---

[1] *Bases of Yoga*, p. 11.
[2] "A quieted mind (not necessarily motionless or silent, though it is good if one can have that at will) and a persistent aspiration in the heart are the two main keys of the Yoga." (*Letters*, Vol. I, p. 311.)
[3] *Letters*, Vol. II, p. 145.
[4] *Bases of Yoga*, p. 2.

disturbs nothing, leaving no trace. Even if a thousand images or the most violent events pass across it, the calm stillness remains as if the very texture of the mind were a substance of eternal and indestructible peace. A mind that has achieved this calmness can begin to act, even intensely and powerfully, but it will keep its fundamental stillness—originating nothing from itself but receiving from Above and giving it a mental form without adding anything of its own, calmly, dispassionately, though with the joy of the Truth and the happy power and light of its passage."[1]

The ability to stand back from the surface activity of the mind; to be the witness and master, rather than the helpless tool of one's thoughts and impressions, is a first step towards this quietude. It may take a long time for the individual finally to break his sense of identity with these surface mental movements and control consciously their acceptance or rejection. To most people their thoughts appear to be intimately linked to their idea of personality; to be in some way a unique expression of what they feel to be themselves and indivisible from consciousness. In the same way they identify themselves with all the other surface movements of their nature, both vital and physical, and have no experience of the true inner being which lies behind them. To break this concentration in the outer nature is of primary importance to the sadhaka.[2]

[1] *Bases of Yoga*, pp. 3-4.
[2] Sri Ramana Maharshi based his *Sadhana* on tireless self-inquiry into the question 'Who am I?' so that this identification with the re-actions and formations of the ego should be laid bare, and the Self ultimately realized. His biographer remarks: "Self-inquiry in daily activity, asking oneself to whom any thought occurs, is a plan of campaign and a very potent one . . . applied to an emotional thought it has terrific potency and strikes at the very root of the passions. One has been hurt and feels resentment—who is hurt or resentful? Who is pleased or despondent, angry or triumphant?" *Ramana Maharshi and the Path of Self-Knowledge*, by Arthur Osborne, p. 153. The Buddhist method of *Satipatthana* has affinities with this technique.

88   FOUNDING THE LIFE DIVINE

In the beginning, peace and calm are rarely continuous. "They come and go," Sri Aurobindo remarks, "and it usually takes a long time to get them settled in the nature."[1] But when quietness comes, keep it and "do not mind if it is for a time an empty quietude; the consciousness is often like a vessel that has to be emptied of its mixed and undesirable contents. . . . The one thing to be avoided is the refilling of the cup with the old turbid contents."[2]

He advises the *sadhaka* to aspire for quietness, peace, calm and to avoid impatience and over-eagerness as this may impair the balance and quiet that has already been achieved. But besides cultivating patience and equability, he also stresses the necessity of avoiding conditions that are liable to draw the aspirant away from inward concentration into the surface consciousness, and the old habitual movements. To take a simple example, he tells a disciple to avoid controversy with people who are antagonistic to the principles of the Yoga. It is not the aspirant's business to convert other people and argument of this kind may draw upon him the adverse forces he is trying to oppose.

Quietness may be imaged as a protective ring encircling the disciple. If he remains within it, he conserves peace and strength instead of dispersing it—as most of us do by unnecessary talk and activity. But if he steps outside the ring or allows it to be invaded by anger or fear, impatience or irritation, he dissolves it and abandons himself to the old clamour and agitation.

In order to keep this inner quietness intact, Sri Aurobindo continually emphasizes the necessity of taking the right attitude—not being influenced in act or judgement by egotism or self-interest; standing back and by detachment achieving an impersonal and impartial view and thus entering into a truer consciousness.

[1] *Bases of Yoga*, p. 11.
[2] Ibid., pp. 9-10.

The wisdom of establishing spiritual experience in the mind and psychic being first is repeatedly stressed by Sri Aurobindo, for a premature descent into, or opening of, the vital being to experience before this is settled in the mind and psychic being may result in great disturbance and confusion. He therefore suggests an initial attempt be made to sense peace above and about the head as a first step. This peace must gradually be experienced as a reality, descending not only into the mind but later on into the vital and physical being.

If conditions are difficult, meet them with equanimity. "Do not be troubled by your surroundings and their opposition," he writes to a disciple. "These conditions are often imposed at first as a kind of ordeal. If you can remain tranquil and undisturbed and continue your sadhana without allowing yourself to be inwardly troubled under these circumstances, it will help to give you a much needed strength."

Again, "there can be no firm foundation in sadhana without equality.[1] Whatever the unpleasantness of circumstances, however disagreeable the conduct of others, you must learn to receive them with a perfect calm and without any disturbing reaction. These things are the test of equality. It is easy to be equal when things go well and circumstances are pleasant; it is when they are the opposite that the completeness of the calm, peace, equality can be tested, reinforced, made perfect."[2]

It is on the ability to achieve quietness, and from quietness, silence, that the aspirant prepares himself for the direct guidance of the Divine in the sadhana. The ordinary life of mind and body—the surface consciousness

[1] Sri Aurobindo follows other translators of the Gita in rendering the word samatā as 'equality'. Equanimity and equability are perhaps better English equivalents and the reader must keep in mind that whenever Sri Aurobindo uses the word equality he intends it in this sense.

[2] Bases of Yoga, pp. 19-20.

in which most people are centred—is always noisy, restless and unpredictable, and it is only by a stilling of this clamour that 'the Voice of intense silence' of which the ancient Hebrews spoke, the voice of the Divine, can begin to be heard at all.

There is naturally considerable difficulty in this first step. The mind is often obstinately and mechanically busy, or, in spite of great activity, it cannot really concentrate at all and wanders; or, if controlled, becomes dull and vacant, not tranquil and lucid. The various methods used for stilling it, given by Sri Aurobindo, will be mentioned later: here we will only add one or two of his general instructions.

Avoid, he says, "fighting with the mind or making mental efforts to pull down the Power or the Silence".[1] Instead, keep only a silent will and aspiration for them. Reject the mind's over-activity without strain or struggle and, above all, do not let depression or despair come in when there is no immediate effect, for this only holds up any progress that is preparing. If the lower vital centre throws up unwelcome formations they must not be accepted, but simply looked at. Refuse sanction to disturbing movements; leave them, by a quiet, persistent, detached refusal, unsupported and unassented to; never consent to ideas, suggestions or feelings that stimulate the old movements that are being supplanted; sanction only peace, calm, purity and whatever else is part of the divine nature.

[1] *Letters*, Vol. II, p. 146.

CHAPTER III

THE LUMINOUS CRYPT OF THE SOUL

When people do sadhana, there is a higher Nature that works within, the psychic and spiritual, and they have to put their natures under the influence of the psychic being and the higher spiritual self or of the Divine.

More Lights on Yoga, p. 27.

The important thing is . . . to live always in the psychic being, your true being. The psychic will, in due time, awaken and turn to the Divine all the rest of the nature, so that even the outer being will feel itself in touch with the Divine and moved by the Divine in all it is and feels and does.

Letters, Vol. I, pp. 228 9.

The psychic is the Divine element in the individual being and its characteristic power is to turn everything towards the Divine.   Ibid., pp. 236–37.

The spiritual conversion begins when the soul begins to insist on a deeper life and is complete when the psychic being becomes the basis or the leader of the consciousness, and mind and vital and body are led by it and obey it.

Ibid., p. 307.

In this Yoga, the psychic being is that which opens the rest of the nature to the true supramental light and finally to the supreme Ananda.   *Lights on Yoga*, p. 32.

It is essential to get back, beyond mind-being, life-being, body-being, still more deeply inward to the psychic entity inmost and profoundest within us—or else to open to the superconscient highest domains. For this penetration into the luminous crypt of the soul one has to get through all the intervening vital stuff to the psychic centre within us, how- ever long, tedious or difficult the process.

The Life Divine, Vol. II (2), p. 935.

THERE are two ways of doing Yoga, says Sri Aurobindo: one is by the action of a vigilant mind which carefully discriminates what is or is not to be done with the help of the Divine Force behind it, the personal effort of the aspirant thereby assuming most of the burden. The other way lies through the opening of the psychic being and its gradual domination of the working of the outer nature through a call for and consent to the Divine action.

In the beginning stages there is nearly always a mixture of these two ways, and indeed, throughout the Yoga the opening of both the heart and mind centres are of primary importance, Sri Aurobindo referring to the nexus between them as the principal means of the attainment.

The heart centre, the seat of the psychic being, is the deepest, as the head is the highest centre.[1] In the chapter on "The Individual Centre" we saw that Sri Aurobindo defines the psychic being as part of the soul. 'Psychic' in this Yoga always refers to the soul, but although Sri Aurobindo occasionally uses the term *psychic being* and *soul* as interchangeable, he generally draws a distinction between them as differently organized parts of the same reality. The psychic being, he writes, does not contain "all that the soul or essential psychic existence bears within it",[2] but it is "formed by the soul in its evolution" and "supports the mind, vital (being), body, grows by their experience, carries the nature from life to life".[3]

In the ordinary man the psychic being is deeply veiled and depends for any expression it may have in his life on the impress it can make through the ordinary mind and vital being, and is therefore subject to their limitations and imperfections. Because it is a spark of the Divine it is in touch with the Force that supports the mind, life and body and is our

---

[1] "These two (the heart centre and the above head—sahasradala—centre) constitute the two poles of the human organism. They are said to be the first centres to form in the embryo, and the terrestrial *prana* (life), derived from the central pranic reservoir in the sun of our planetary system, is said to direct their formation." (The Tibetan *Book of the Dead,* p. 217.) "The centre which opens directly to the Self is above the head, altogether outside the physical body, in what is called the subtle body, *śukṣma śarīra.*" (*Lights on Yoga,* p. 36.)

[2] *Letters,* Vol. I, p. 141.

[3] Ibid., pp. 144-5.

nearest and surest means of guidance. It can feel the Divine easily and swiftly, once it is awake, and, once awakened, it makes no mistakes, so that its tutelage is infallible.

The mind and vital being on the contrary can confuse other suggestions for the Divine will. "The mind has its ideas and clings to them," Sri Aurobindo states, "the human vital (being) resists surrender, for what it calls surrender in the early stages is a doubtful kind of self-giving with a demand in it; the physical consciousness is like a stone and what it calls surrender is often no more than inertia. It is only the psychic (being) that knows how to surrender and the psychic (being) is usually very much veiled in the beginning. When the psychic (being) awakes, it can bring a sudden and true surrender of the whole being, for the difficulty of the rest is rapidly dealt with and disappears. But till then effort is indispensable."[1]

The psychic being, then, is our inmost being. Its seat is not above the head, as that of the Self, but behind the heart. Sri Aurobindo characterizes its power as "not knowledge but an essential or spiritual feeling—it has the clearest sense of the Truth and a sort of inherent perception of it". It does not analyse or experiment but "seeks, feels, experiences".[2] Its nature is one of simple, spontaneous self-giving without reservation or ulterior motive, in contrast to the mental and vital beings, which always hope to get some private gratification out of the Yoga, or only surrender themselves conditionally.

The heart is the centre of the highest part of the emotional being. It is also the centre where the mind and higher vital meet, the psychic being standing behind them. To reach it necessitates a deep plunge inward, for it must not be confused with the inner mental, vital and physical being, as it is even more inward in nature.

Each of us, so long as we remain bound to the con-

[1] *Lights on Yoga*, p. 27.
Letters, Vol. II, p. 100.

ditions of what Sri Aurobindo terms 'the Ignorance' (*avidyā*), imagines our central being to be the ordinary mental, vital or physical consciousness—whichever happens to be the plane on which we live predominantly—and we talk glibly about our souls when, in actuality, we have absolutely no true or direct experience of them. Truly, most of us, in Matthew Arnold's words, "never once possess our soul Before we die".

The great importance of bringing forward the psychic being, so that it may impose its change on all the outer nature, is that its response to the Divine is pure and steadfast. It refuses to be deceived or taken in and immediately discriminates between right and wrong movements. Though its control is at first very imperfect it gains strength every time there is a higher movement in us. Its actual effect on the development of the Yoga is decisive, for its opening and perfect control over the nature is the preliminary to the Divine guidance itself.

The results in the *sadhana* of this realization and opening of the psychic being are manifold. Sri Aurobindo stipulates two things as being necessary for the discovery of true individuality. One is the realization of the psychic being; the other is the conscious detachment of the soul (*purusha*) from the nature (*prakriti*), that is, from the working of the external life of mind and body with which the soul habitually identifies itself.

Of the two methods of opening to the Divine—through the heart centre and the psychic being, or through the mind centres and the higher consciousness—he always favours the first method, though he is never dogmatic, stating that different natures require different approaches. He prefers the concentration in the heart[1] for a number

[1] Those familiar with the psychology of Mahayana Buddhism will remember significantly that the heart centre is the seat of the Buddha Amitabha, 'He of Boundless Light', the Illuminator and Enlightener, whose 'radiant light-path' is that of Discriminating Wisdom. He is one of the five Dhyani Buddhas who symbolize progression from bondage to freedom.

of reasons, one being that for the majority of people it is the easiest, the opening in the head, either through the forehead centre or 'the thousand-petalled lotus' above the head, presenting too difficult an opening for many aspirants. But there are other reasons. Difficulties are reduced to the minimum once the psychic being can be brought to the front "and pour its influence on all the movements of the mind, the vital and the physical consciousness";[1] for though the work of transformation has still to be done, it will no longer be so dry and painful.

The psychic being always brings with it light and happiness and peace; also an intensity of aspiration and a deep and true desire for surrender. Its attributes are a perception of the truth and a sense of the Divine and an unfailing discernment of what is good. Its realization brings "Bhakti, self-giving, surrender, turning of all the movements Godward, discrimination and choice of all that belongs to the Divine Truth, Good, Beauty, rejection of all that is false, evil, ugly, discordant, union through love and sympathy with all existence, openness to the Truth of the Self and the Divine".[2] It leads to a quieting and purification of the mind, vital and physical consciousness, embracing everything requisite, "right thought, right perception, right feeling, right attitude".[3]

Therefore, the more the heart centre is open and the soul in front and active, "the quicker, safer, easier the working of the Force can be".[4] The psychic being will always reveal egotistical traits. Its power is that of dismissing instantly all things foreign to its nature or which pull the consciousness down. By its realization the aspirant becomes aware of his soul and no longer identifies himself with his mental or vital being.

---

[1] *More Lights on Yoga*, p. 84.
[2] *Letters*, Vol. I, p. 147.
[3] Ibid., p. 155.
[4] *Lights on Yoga*, p. 38.

There is another reason why Sri Aurobindo advocates the opening of the heart centre first. The descent of the higher consciousness, and the transformation of the nature at which the Yoga aims, become safer and easier through the bringing forward of the psychic being and its preparation of the mental, vital and physical consciousness.

As we have mentioned before, he continually stresses the dangers latent in a descent of power, even of the purest kind, into a nature where any traces of egotism remain, and probably there is not a single aspirant who has not at some time encountered individuals shipwrecked in this way.[1]

The method of the psychic being is to smooth the road. "When the psychic (being) is in front" (he writes), "the sadhana becomes natural and easy and it is only a question of time and natural development. When the mind or the vital or the physical consciousness is on top, then the sadhana is a tapasya[2] and a struggle."[3]

This realization is of such vital importance in Integral Yoga that Sri Aurobindo comes back to it again and again in his teaching to his disciples, emphasizing that there can be no conversion without the awakening of the psychic being.

What methods are we to use in endeavouring to open the heart centre and what are the indications which entitle the aspirant to know when it has been achieved?

Concerning the first point, Sri Aurobindo carefully distinguishes the conditions and methods necessary for liberating the psychic being, saying that it is only possible to open it fully when "the sadhak has got rid of the mixture of vital motives with his sadhana and is capable of a

[1] There are great resources of pranic energies in the vital centres (navel and abdominal), and if the Force pours in through the head centres and floods the vital while it is still impure, such things as anger, sex, fear, doubt, will be stirred into activity and rush up and cloud the mind (cf. *More Lights on Yoga*, p. 51. *Bases of Yoga*, pp. 87-91).
[2] *Tapasya*: spiritual effort by special discipline or process.
[3] *Letters*, Vol. IV, p. 174.

simple and sincere self-offering. . . . If there is any kind of egoistic turn or insincerity of motive, if the Yoga is done under a pressure of vital demands, or partly or wholly to satisfy some spiritual or other ambition, pride, vanity or seeking after power, position or influence over others or with any push towards satisfying any vital desire with the help of the Yogic force, then the psychic (being) cannot open, or opens only partially or only at times and shuts again because it is veiled by the vital smoke. Also, if the mind takes the leading part in the Yoga and puts the soul into the background, or, if the bhakti or other movements of the sadhana take more of a vital than of a psychic form, there is the same inability. Purity, simple sincerity and the capacity of an unegoistic unmixed self-offering without pretension or demand are the condition of an entire opening of the psychic being."[1]

This opening is greatly facilitated, not only when the egocentricity is much diminished, but also when there is a strong devotion for the Divine, humility, and a sense of submission and dependence.

The method he advocates is concentration in the heart.[2] This concentration opens within; through it one becomes aware of the soul, the divine element in the individual. As we have seen, once it can begin to come forward and govern the nature, it will turn the latter in all its movements towards the Divine. This concentration should be accompanied by an aspiration for the Presence in the heart and for the inward opening, the main supports of this part of the sadhana being "aspiration, prayer, bhakti, love, surrender . . . accompanied by a rejection of all that stands in the way of what we aspire for".[3]

[1] Lights on Yoga, pp. 29-30.
[2] "There is no method in this Yoga except to concentrate, preferably in the heart, and call the presence of the Mother (the Divine Shakti) to take up the being and by the workings of her force transform the consciousness." (Bases of Yoga, p. 29.)
[3] Lights on Yoga, p. 39.

98 FOUNDING THE LIFE DIVINE

Again, "aspiration, constant and sincere, and the will
to turn to the Divine alone are the best means to bring
forward the psychic (being)".[1] Quietude, peace and silence
in the heart and vital being (which the heart commands)
are essential, and a mind free from mental constructions,
filled only with devotion and self-giving to the Divine.

Confusion must not be made between the *inner being*
and the *psychic being*. The former refers to the true mental,
true vital, true physical being, which ordinarily remains
veiled and silent behind the mental, vital and physical
ego.[2] To reach it and to know it also requires a deep going
inward, but the psychic being, influencing the consciousness from behind, is deeper still.

In order to reach this hidden seat of the soul the
aspirant has first to pass through the inner, or true,
mental, vital and physical being. "It is absolutely necessary for our purpose," Sri Aurobindo states, "that one
should become conscious in these inner regions, for if they
are not awake, then the psychic being has no proper and
sufficient instrumentation for its activities; it has only the
outer mind, outer vital (being) and body for its means and
these are small and narrow and obscure."[3] And in another
place he writes: "Each time there is a purification of the
outer nature, it becomes more possible for the inner being
to reveal itself, to become free and to open to the higher
consciousness above."[4]

Awareness of this inner being when it rises to meet the
higher consciousness is sometimes felt as an inward detaching and floating upward; to pass into the inner being is
often accompanied by a tendency to lose consciousness of
the outer world, called *samadhi* or Yoga-trance.

---

[1] *Letters*, Vol. II, p. 98.
[2] "The inner consciousness means the inner mind, inner vital, inner
physical and behind them the psychic which is their inmost being."
(*Letters*, Vol. I, p. 163.)
[3] Ibid., p. 161.
[4] Ibid., p. 224.

The beginning of psychic awareness may be accompanied by a sense of division; a feeling, necessary to Yogic development but sometimes puzzling, of housing "a twofold being, the inner psychic which is the true one and the other, the outer human being which is instrumental for the outward life".[1] There is nothing wrong in this experience, Sri Aurobindo tells us, it is indispensable and normal at this stage. The important thing is "to keep what you have and let it grow, to live always in the psychic being, your true being".[2] In time even the outer nature will feel the Divine Presence and live and move in it.

To imagine that this realization is soon or easily come by would be a great mistake. The direct action of the psychic being appears only at a high stage of individual development or by Yoga, and without experienced discrimination it is easy to mistake the intuitions of the inner being for its guidance. It is marked by what Sri Aurobindo calls a psychic discrimination; by a power of constant intimation from within; and finally by a control which illumines and patiently removes all imperfections, mental, vital and physical. Again, he says that awareness of the psychic being starts when the inmost knowledge begins to come and we have ceased to identify ourselves with the vital or mental formations of our being. Until then we must continue to put forward a strong but calm personal effort in trying to fulfil the initial stages of the sadhana; remain vigilant and obediently follow the counsel of the Master or Teacher.

[1] Letters, Vol. I, p. 228.
[2] Ibid., Vol. I, p. 228.

CHAPTER IV

WORK, MEDITATION AND CONCENTRATION

All work done for the Divine, from poetry and art and music to carpentry or baking or sweeping a room, should be made perfect even in its smallest external detail as well as in the spirit in which it is done; for only then is it an altogether fit offering.

Letters, Vol. III (On Poetry and Literature), p. 290.

I mean by work action done for the Divine and more and more in union with the Divine—for the Divine alone and nothing else. Naturally that is not easy at the beginning, any more than deep meditation and luminous knowledge are easy or even true love and bhakti are easy. But like the others it has to be begun in the right spirit and attitude, with the right will in you, then all the rest will come.

Lights on Yoga, p. 52.

The only work that spiritually purifies is that which is done without personal motives, without desire for fame or public recognition or worldly greatness, without insistence on one's own mental motives or vital lusts and demands or physical preferences, without vanity or crude self-assertion or claim for position or prestige, done for the sake of the Divine alone and at the command of the Divine. All work done in an egoistic spirit, however good for people in the world of the Ignorance, is of no avail to the seeker of the Yoga.

Ibid., pp. 46-7.

It is so that life can be changed into worship, by putting behind it the spirit of a transcendent and universal love, the seeking of oneness, the sense of oneness; by making each act a symbol, and expression of Godward emotion or a relation with the Divine; by turning all we do into an act of worship, an act of the soul's communion, the mind's understanding, the life's obedience, the heart's surrender.

The Synthesis of Yoga, p. 139.

I

THE NECESSITY FOR A THREE-FOLD BASE

IN DISCUSSING the question of works and meditation in Sri Aurobindo's teaching, we must keep in mind that Integral Yoga is founded on (though not limited by) the *Karma Yoga* of the *Gita*, a system of spiritual discipline, in Sri Aurobindo's own words, which takes work (dedicated to the Divine) as its basis. It is also a Yoga of love and knowledge as well as of action. Indeed, its burthen is that man cannot act in truth until he has found the ground of Truth and established it as the centre of his consciousness; and this he may do only with the aid of Knowledge and Love, which lead him to the Highest.

For Sri Aurobindo, concerned with the terrestrial consciousness and founding a divine life in the world, the external life is the acid test of the inner life created by Integral Yoga. This is not because there can be no realization of God without such an outward perfecting. There have been many God-realized men, he points out, whose inner development had little or no effect on their outer nature and who remained rude, bad-tempered or hostile in their relationships with the world.

Those who choose a life of world-negating spirituality may concentrate on the inner realization and disregard the external nature. But Integral Yoga is concerned with life and the world and demands something fuller than the 'Mary-consciousness' which distinguishes such a way. It is a descent as well as an ascent of consciousness, therefore it must untie and not cut every Gordian knot it encounters.

If there is no transformation of the stubborn resistances of the outer nature, no ultimate descent of the light into the dense, obstinate subconscient levels of the physical nature, there is no *integral* Yoga in the full sense in which this word is meant by Sri Aurobindo, because for this the aspirant "must have the same consciousness in inner experience and outward action".[1]

Love and knowledge are naturally gathered into its practice as vital elements. "The self-offering to the Divine, the consecration of oneself to the Divine which is the essence of this *Karma Yoga* are essentially a movement of bhakti," he states, "only it (Integral Yoga) does exclude a life-fleeing exclusive meditation[2] or an emotional bhakti shut up in its own inner dream taken as the whole movement of the Yoga. One may have hours of pure absorbed meditation or of the inner motionless adoration and ecstasy, but they are not the whole of the Integral Yoga."[3] And again he exclaims trenchantly to an inquirer: "How are you going to find the right external relations by withdrawing altogether from external relations? And how do you propose to be thoroughly transformed and unified by living only in the internal life, without any test of the transformation and unity by external contact and the ordeals of the external work and life? Thoroughness includes external work and relations and not a retired inner life only."[4]

In another instance he insists that though trance

---

[1] *Lights on Yoga*, p. 45.

[2] In this essentially life-affirming spiritual philosophy, Sri Aurobindo will always substitute the idea of *right use* for renunciation wherever possible. For instance, the problem of wealth and of money is not solved in any way by taking vows of poverty, excepting in a limited individual sense. "Some even put a ban on money and riches," he writes in *The Mother* (p. 22 passim.), "and proclaim poverty and bareness of life as the only spiritual condition. But that is an error; it leaves the power in the hands of the hostile forces. To reconquer it for the Divine to whom it belongs and use it divinely for the divine life is the supramental way for the Sadhaka. . . . In your personal use of money look on all you have or get or bring as the Mother's (the Divine *Shakti's*). Make no demand but accept what you receive from her and use it for the purposes for which it is given to you. Be entirely selfless, entirely scrupulous, exact, careful in detail, a good trustee; always consider that it is her possessions and not your own that you are handling."

[3] *Lights on Yoga*, p. 53.

[4] *More Lights on Yoga*, p. 50.

(*samadhi*) has utility in opening the being and preparing it, all experience of realization must also come and endure in the waking state to be truly possessed. "If experienced in trance," he states, "it will be a superconscient state only for some part of the inner being but not real to the whole consciousness. . . . Therefore in this Yoga much value is given to the waking realization and experience." Again, "the including of the outer consciousness in the transformation is of supreme importance in the Yoga— meditation cannot do it. Meditation can deal only with the inner being. So work is of primary importance—only it must be done with the right attitude and in the right consciousness, then it is as fruitful as any meditation can be."[1] If we may translate into Western terms, in this Yoga Mary *and* Martha must be in every soul.

Because of its greater applicability to the majority of aspirants; the greater facility with which most people can use its methods—as compared, for instance, with meditation—and also because of its simplicity, Sri Aurobindo therefore gives a good deal of attention to the place of work in the Yoga. But it must be stressed that he does not over-emphasize its importance in the *sadhana* at the expense of devotion and meditation. "I have stressed both bhakti and knowledge in my Yoga as well as works," he has said, "even if I have not given any of them an exclusive importance."[2]

II

WORK

Work is not only a means of serving the Divine and testing the values of the inner life; a certain amount of it is also necessary for the proper balance of the being. "A

[1] *Letters*, Vol. II, p. 9.
[2] *Lights on Yoga*, p. 50.

complete cessation of work and entire withdrawal into oneself is seldom advisable," Sri Aurobindo writes, "it may encourage a too one-sided and visionary condition in which one lives in a sort of mid-world of purely subjective experiences without a firm hold on either external reality or on the highest Reality and without the right use of the subjective experience to create a firm link and then a unification between the highest Reality and the external realization in life."[1]

Work done "for the Divine alone and nothing else", as the *Gita* teaches, can be, he says, as effective as devotion and contemplation. By rejecting all forms of egoism and desire one gets "a quietude and purity into which the Peace ineffable can descend; one gets by the dedication of one's will in the Divine Will the death of ego and the enlarging into the cosmic consciousness or else the uplifting into what is above the cosmic. ... By constant referring of all one's will and works to the Divine, love and adoration grow, the psychic being comes forward. By the reference to the Power above, we can come to feel it above and its descent and the opening to an increasing consciousness and knowledge. Finally, works, bhakti and knowledge go together and self-perfection becomes possible—what we call the transformation of the nature".[2]

The same Force that works through meditation can also act through, support and guide work executed in the right spirit, provided the *sadhak* learns to open to it; but this means doing it "well and carefully as a sacrifice to the Divine, without desire or egoism, with equality of mind and calm tranquillity in good or bad fortune, for the sake of the Divine and not for the sake of any personal gain, reward or result, with the consciousness that it is the Divine Power to which all work belongs".[3]

[1] *Lights on Yoga*, p. 59.
[2] Ibid., pp. 52-3.
[3] Ibid., p. 47.

Work done in this spirit is "a powerful means of sadhana and . . . such work is especially necessary in this Yoga".[1] And by work Sri Aurobindo means *all* work that is not in its nature undivine, whether intellectual or physical work. The idea that physical work is inferior to mental culture, he states, springs from the arrogant pretensions of the intellect. Not only is all work done for the Divine equally divine, but manual labour done for the Divine is more divine than mental culture done for one's own sake.

How can the aspirant best begin to practise this opening in work that will culminate in "the automatic constant realization of Yoga, divine union, in works"?[2]

There are two main places where the consciousness can be centred for Yoga, in the heart and in the head—the soul-centre and the mind-centre. The former, it will be remembered, opens inward to the psychic being and the Presence in the heart. Few people can hope at first to be made aware of this presence of the Divine all the time, or even intermittently, but it should be aspired for and practised from the earliest stages.

Begin, Sri Aurobindo advises, by remembering and dedicating the work when it is taken up and give thanks at the end. Practise recollection when there is a pause; aspire for the assistance of the Divine or to be made aware of the supporting Presence. Concentrate in the heart and "call the presence and power of the Mother to take up the being and by the workings of her force transform the consciousness".[3]

If you cannot remember the Divine all the time while you are working, he tells a disciple, it does not greatly matter. "When people remember all the time during work (it can be done), it is usually with the back of their minds

[1] *Letters*, Vol. II, p. 16.
[2] *Lights on Yoga*, p. 46.
[3] *Bases of Yoga*, p. 29.

or else there is created gradually a faculty of double
thought or else a double consciousness—one in front that
works, and one within that witnesses and remembers.
There is also another way which was mine for a long time
—a condition in which the work takes place automatically
and without intervention of personal thought or mental
action, while the consciousness remains silent in the
Divine. The thing, however, does not come so much by
trying as by a very simple constant aspiration and will of
concentration—or else by a movement of the consciousness separating the inner from the instrumental being.
Aspiration and will of consecration calling down a greater
Force to do the work is a method which brings great
results, even if it takes a long time about it. That is a great
secret of sadhana, to know how to get things done by the
Power behind or above instead of doing all by the mind's
effort."[1]

Again, he says that while there should be no meditation at the time of work, for this would withdraw the
attention, "there should be the constant memory of the
One to whom you offer it", until this gives way to a constant experience "of a calm being within concentrated in
the sense of the Divine Presence while the surface mind
does the work".[2]

In another place, writing of the right attitude in work,
he states: "The ideal state for work is when there is a
natural concentration of the consciousness in the special
energy, supported by an easeful rest and quiescence of the
consciousness as a whole. Distraction of the mind by other
activities disturbs this balance of ease and concentrated
energy—fatigue also disturbs or destroys it. . . . The best
expenditure of energy is that which flows easily without
effort at all—when the inspiration or Force (any Force)
works of itself and the mind and vital (being) and even

[1] *Lights on Yoga*, pp. 50-1.
[2] Ibid., p. 46.

the body are glowing instruments and the Force flows out in an intense and happy working—an almost labourless labour."[1]

This practice of the Presence of God in work can only be perfected by constant endeavour; patience and resolution, Sri Aurobindo has counselled, are needed in every method of the *sadhana*. The necessity of *apramatta*[2] disappears, he writes, only when the memory of the Yoga and its objects can be replaced by the continual remembrance of God in all things and happenings.

Work by itself, he adds, is only a preparation, as meditation is only a preparation. Both are an equal means of realization and it would be a grave error to suppose that major realizations may not come through work done in an increasing Yogic consciousness: many have had them by this means.

III

MEDITATION AND CONCENTRATION

In Yoga, concentration is either located in a particular place or aims at a gathered condition throughout the whole being. The method we have been discussing is primarily concerned with achieving an opening through the heart-centre, while meditation and concentration, in the mind-centres, aims at an opening either through the forehead-centre or the centre above the head.

Sri Aurobindo has many things to say about the opening through the head. He calls it "a too difficult opening"[3] for many people, advocating by preference, for the foundation of this particular Yoga, the concentration in the heart, which is designed to open directly to the safe

---

[1] *Letters*, Vol. I, pp. 239-41.
[2] *Apramatta*: being without negligence, not losing oneself.
[3] *Bases of Yoga*, p. 29.

guidance of the soul. "This Yoga too is not a Yoga of knowledge alone, knowledge is one of its means, but its base being self-offering, surrender, bhakti, it is based in the heart and nothing can be eventually done without this base."[1]

In the case of his own disciples he observes: "There are plenty of people here who do or have done Japa and base themselves on bhakti, very few comparatively who have done the 'head' meditation; love and bhakti and works are usually the base; how many can proceed by knowledge? Only the few."[2]

In another place he remarks: "Meditation is one means of approach to the Divine and a great way, but it cannot be called a short cut—for most it is a long and most difficult though a very high ascent. . . . It is very indispensable but there is nothing of the short cut about it."[3] Provided they do not take on too vital a character, he states, the only short cuts to the Divine are love, bhakti, surrender and the psychic opening.

Meditation may seem to the novice the one, indispensable technique of the contemplative life, but on the contrary, Sri Aurobindo says, it is only one method for calling down the true consciousness. The most important thing is to feel the descent of this true consciousness and to join with it; if it happens to come—as it did in his own case—without the orthodox method, so much the better. Meditation is only a device, he reminds us; the true movement is to remain in *sadhana* whatever one is doing, working, talking, acting.

In some cases, Sri Aurobindo advised disciples not to meditate at all. It would therefore appear that for certain people in the early stages its practice is inadvisable or unsuitable.

[1] *Letters*, Vol. II, p. 12.
[2] Ibid.
[3] Ibid., p. 13.

Nevertheless, meditation, together with bhakti and works is one of the main supports of the Yoga. The aspirant may use all three, or two, or only one. In time the practice of one will bring in all the rest. To open to the Divine Influence is the cardinal necessity in this Yoga and each must choose the method which suits him best. Everyone has his, or her, own way of treading the path and some find the head concentration easiest, others the concentration in the heart; some can do both, for it is inevitable that the *sadhana* should combine the two approaches in some measure, but "to begin with the heart-centre, if one can do it," Sri Aurobindo advises, "is the more desirable".[1] "The more love and bhakti and surrender grow in the heart," he says elsewhere, "the more rapid and perfect becomes the evolution of the sadhana."[2]

He defines meditation and concentration in these words: "Concentration means fixing the consciousness in one place or on one object and in a single condition. Meditation can be diffusive, e.g. thinking about the Divine, receiving impressions and discriminating, watching what goes on in the nature and acting upon it, etc."[3] But, as he points out in another context, "aspiration, prayer, concentration, intensity" are all a natural part of meditation, all being designed to lead eventually to union.

Concentration should be quiet and steady, without over-eagerness or violence of effort. Whether centred in the heart or the head, it does not mean keeping the attention fixed on a particular spot. The aspirant must take "a station of consciousness in either place and concentrate there not on the place, but on the Divine".[4] If the concentration is concerned with thought, then it will be in one of the head-centres; if with the feeling, in the heart.

[1] *Letters*, Vol. I, p. 75.
[2] *Lights on Yoga*, p. 38.
[3] *Letters*, Vol. II, p. 144.
[4] *More Lights on Yoga*, p. 97.

It can be done with eyes opened or closed, whichever is preferred. Concentration in the heart should be a call to the Divine to manifest there; it should be supported by aspiration, prayer, bhakti, love, surrender and a rejection of all that stands in the way of the *sadhana*.

The mind-centres open to the higher consciousness and concentration there is accompanied by "an aspiration and call and a sustained will for the descent of the Divine Peace, Power, Light, Knowledge, Ananda into the being —the Peace first or the Peace and Force together. Some indeed," he adds, "receive Light first or Ananda first or some sudden pouring down of knowledge."[1]

This concentration may be aided, if the *sadhaka* wishes, by using with it one of the disciplinary processes of the old Yogas.[2] One may concentrate on a word, a name, an idea, an image, or a combination of these things. For example, one may concentrate on the idea of the Divine; on a Figure of Light such as Christ or the Buddha, or a Master; on the word *Om*;[3] on the idea of Peace; or on a short sentence such as "Be still and know that I am God", "Come for refuge to Me alone".

If concentrating in the time-honoured place between the eyebrows,[4] the centre of the inner mind, Sri Aurobindo

[1] *Lights on Yoga*, p. 39.
[2] I.e. the *Advaita* process by which the aspirant rejects identification with the mind, vital being, body, saying: "I am not the mind. I am not the vital being," etc. Or the method of the *Sankhyas*, the separation of *Prakriti* from *Purusha*—outer nature from the soul. (*Lights on Yoga*, p. 40.) Practice of the four Brahma-Viharas (Loving-Kindness, Compassion, Sympathetic Joy, Equanimity) of Buddhism are also helpful. The disciplines that involve special breathing of a very intensive kind should be avoided by those not directly under the guidance of a Master, as they may damage the subtle bodies or disturb their balance.
[3] *Om*: The primal sound representing the supreme spiritual reality. (*Lights on Yoga*, p. 56.)
[4] The location of this centre is actually in the middle of the forehead. It is sometimes called the third eye because its development brings the power of inner vision.

says: "Think firmly from there on whatever you make the object of your concentration or else try to see the image of it from there. If you succeed in this, then after a time you feel that your whole consciousness is centred there in that place—of course for the time being. After doing it for some time and often it becomes easy and normal."[1]

To concentrate too long before one is accustomed causes fatigue and this should be avoided. Instead of concentrating one can relax and meditate. Deep concentration and meditation should only be done when the aspirant is alone and quiet. Sometimes, in the early stages of meditation, the pressure to go inside, into a deep inner consciousness, is mistaken by the mind for a pressure to go to sleep. This tendency to sleep is often a first difficulty, but with perseverance, Sri Aurobindo writes, the sleep changes to an inner conscious state.

The concentration in the forehead-centre should always be looked upon as a preparation for the consciousness to rise to the station above (*sahasradala chakra*). Otherwise, Sri Aurobindo states, "one may get shut up in one's own mind and its experiences or at best attain only to a reflection of the Truth above instead of rising into the spiritual transcendence to live there".[2]

Neither concentration nor meditation can be done without a quietening of the outer mind. Most people are acutely aware, when they first begin to practise these things, of the extreme liveliness of their own thoughts, over which they have singularly little control.

We dealt with some of these problems in the chapter on 'The Quiet Mind' and Sri Aurobindo makes further references to the question of stilling the mind in his teaching on meditation and concentration. Direct efforts to still the mind are a difficult method, he writes; the best way is to gain the psychic control, which, when it spreads in

[1] *Lights on Yoga*, p. 43.
[2] *Letters*, Vol. I, p. 74.

the outer being, quietens the mechanical activity of the subconscious mind.

The buzz of the physical mind should be rejected quietly and without disturbance, until it slackens for want of encouragement. There are always two things, he says, which can rise up and assail the silence: suggestions from the vital being and the physical mind's mechanical recurrences. Calm rejection is the cure for both.

The soul can control the lower nature, but its will is a quiet one; any perturbation or agitation over difficulties prevents the will of the soul from acting as effectively as it would otherwise.

In another place, writing on silencing the mind, he observes that the problem is not so much getting rid of mental activity as converting it into the right thing.[1] Doing nothing with the mind is not quiet or silence, for it is inactivity that keeps the mind working mechanically and discursively, while concentration, by gathering it into a focal point, steadies and quiets it. "If the mind is active," Sri Aurobindo writes, "one has to learn to look at it, drawn back and not giving any sanction from within, until its habitual or mechanical activities begin to fall quiet for want of support from within."[2]

Silence does not, however, mean absence of experiences. It is a quietude in which experiences can take place without causing any disturbances. As we have seen, Sri Aurobindo discourages all methods which involve struggle or strain, or wrestling with the mind to quiet it, for usually the mind comes out victorious from the battle.

"It is this standing back, detaching oneself, getting

[1] Sri Aurobindo states his case for the Affirmative Way in these words: "The negative means are not evil; they are useful for their object which is to get away from life. But from the positive point of view they are disadvantageous, because they get rid of the powers of the being instead of divinizing them for the transformation of life." (*More Lights on Yoga*, pp. 96-7.)
[2] *Letters*, Vol. II, p. 146.

the power to listen to something other than the thoughts of the external mind that is the easier way," he writes. "At the same time one can look up, as it were, imaging to oneself the Force as there just above and calling it down or quietly expecting its help. That is how most people do it, till the mind falls gradually quiet or silent of itself, or else silence begins to descend from above."[1]

Remain quiet at the time of meditation, he advises; do not fight with the mind or make mental efforts to pull down the Power or the Silence, but keep only a silent will and aspiration for them.

While concentration entails a gathering together of consciousness at one point, or a gathered condition throughout the whole being, the process of meditation may be different. "It is not indispensable to gather like this," Sri Aurobindo observes, "one can simply remain with a quiet mind thinking of one subject for (the purpose of) observing what comes in the consciousness and dealing with it."[2] This method necessitates restfully opening to the Force so that it may work peacefully and freely in the *adhara*.

To spend excessive energy in prayer or meditation or spiritual practice of this intensive kind is a strain even to those accomplished in these methods. Also, the attempt to break down the walls between the inner and the outer self by strenuous meditation or by what Sri Aurobindo calls "certain methods of tense endeavour", before completing the preliminary stages of the *sadhana*, may lead to conditions which may be "very turbid, chaotic, beset with unnecessary dangers".[3]

Any pulling down of the Force, for the inexperienced, either by this kind of violent effort or by the wrong kind of desire, is not safe. "Not safe," comments Sri Auro-

[1] *Letters*, Vol. II, pp. 145-6.
[2] Ibid., pp. 143-4.
[3] Ibid, Vol. I, p. 212.

bindo, "first, because it may lead to violent reactions, or it brings down contrary or wrong or mixed forces which the sadhaka is not experienced enough to distinguish from the true ones. Or else it may substitute the sadhaka's own limited power of experience or his mental and vital constructions for the free gift and true leading of the Divine. Cases differ, each has his own way of sadhana."[1]

The natural posture for concentrated meditation is the sitting motionless position. Yogis always sit in an *āsana* (posture); for example, the famous lotus position in which seated Buddhas are depicted, with the feet drawn up on the thighs. Some Westerners can sit in this position without difficulty or in a modified version of it like the Buddhist 'Sukh'āsana'; others can learn it, but to most people, unused to sitting from childhood on the floor, like the Indians, it is not at all easy. It is not necessary to adopt this position, though if it comes naturally it is the most gathered, comfortable and poised.

The most important thing is to keep the neck and spine in a straight line.[2] If the hands are lightly clasped and the feet placed together, this closes the circuit and prevents the escape of energy from the body. Meditation can also be practised lying down, but this position is inclined to be too passive. Those who have a settled quietude in the consciousness can concentrate and receive experiences while walking or in an active condition, but for the beginner the gathered posture of sitting motionless is the best.

To digress a moment from Sri Aurobindo's teaching, it would seem that the chronic inability of Westerners to relax creates a special difficulty for them in the practice of meditation. Owing to the important psycho-physiological

[1] *Bases of Yoga*, p. 42.
[2] Again, cases differ, and it would be unwise to be dogmatic even on this point. In *Heaven and You* W. Macmillan states that he is able to meditate sitting relaxed in a chair and without adopting any of the traditional postures.

relation between tension and the activity of thinking, any tendency to muscular tension must help to stimulate the physical mind, and this is to be avoided.

Some people may therefore find it an assistance to relax thoroughly for five minutes, or more if necessary, before attempting to meditate. By this is meant a careful and disciplined attempt to make every part of the body relax, starting from the crown of the head (scalp), eyes, root of tongue, back of neck, jaw, and so on, down to the toes. Deep breathing is an aid to relaxation, and is often a help in controlling nervousness.

There is no fixed *japa* or *mantra*[1] in this Yoga, and no stress is laid on their use, though Sri Aurobindo is not against their adoption by anyone finding them helpful. "The stress is rather on an aspiration in the consciousness and a concentration of the mind, heart, will, all the being," he writes.[2]

Lastly, to those with the aptitude, Sri Aurobindo encourages the continuation of all creative activity, such as composing, painting, writing poetry, for these things give the experience of living in the inner being. They help and do not hinder the inner preparation, being a means of developing the right position of receptivity and bringing out the *bhakti* which is there in the inner being. But to this he adds a word of warning: "Every artist (there are rare exceptions) has got something of the public man in him, in his vital-physical parts, the need of the stimulus of an audience, social applause, satisfied vanity or fame. That must go absolutely if he wants to be a Yogi and his art a service not of man or of his own ego but of the Divine."[3]

---

[1] *Japa*: repetition of set sounds or words or a name as prayer or invocation. *Mantra*: set words or sounds having a spiritual significance and power. (*More Lights on Yoga*, pp. 137-8)
[2] *Letters*, Vol. I, p. 247.
[3] *More Lights on Yoga*, p. 44.

CHAPTER V

IN DIFFICULTY

The goal of Yoga is always hard to reach, but this one is more difficult than any other, and it is only for those who have the call, the capacity to face everything and every risk, even the risk of failure, and the will to progress towards an entire selflessness, desirelessness and surrender.
Bases of Yoga, pp. 69–70.

The road of Yoga is long, and every inch of ground has to be won against much resistance, and no quality is more needed by the sadhaka than patience and single-minded perseverance with a faith that remains firm through all difficulties, delays and apparent failures. Ibid., p. 46.

The world will trouble you so long as any part of you belongs to the world. It is only if you belong entirely to the Divine that you can become free. Ibid., p. 68.

This Yoga is a spiritual battle; its very attempt raises all sorts of adverse forces, and one must be ready to face difficulties, sufferings, reverses of all sorts in a calm and unflinching spirit. *Letters*, Vol. IV, p. 376.

The spiritual change which Yoga demands from human nature and individual character is . . . full of difficulties, one may almost say that it is the most difficult of all human aspirations and efforts. *Letters*, Vol. I, p. 288.

I

THE CHARACTERISTIC DIFFICULTIES OF YOGA

ALL Yogas without exception are difficult, Sri Aurobindo once wrote in a letter, and though a few great souls prepared by past lives may attain the goal more swiftly, for most people it lies at the end of a long and difficult endeavour. Of all Yogas it can be said "Difficult is that road, hard to tread like the edge of a razor."[1]

In so arduous an undertaking as the total spiritual transformation of the nature it is inevitable that the way should often be strewn with obstacles of every kind. If it were not so, he observes, it would be a multitude and not simply a minority of aspirants that would be practising Yoga, and he reminds us that not even a Christ or a Buddha has been without doubts and despairs. If Yoga is neither safe nor easy, neither is ordinary life, in which sorrows, difficulties and disasters continue to the end and where the individual is not only unable to find any release from them, but is often without the support of faith which sustains the *sadhaka* with the consolation that he is moving surely towards a serenity which outer disturbances may still touch but not trouble.

Bright and dark periods are universal in *sadhana*. They are the 'day and night' of the Vedic seers. For most people, though not for all, the dry periods lie at the beginning and lessen gradually. To be prepared for some of the difficulties with which we may be faced and to know the right attitude to take with them is of immense assistance in lessening the hardships of these ordeals. Sri Aurobindo deals at great length with this subject and in order to make the maximum use of all the help he gives us in the many problems with which it confronts us, it would be well to begin by looking at some of the more general dangers and difficulties which we may expect to encounter.

In the second volume of his published *Letters*, Sri Aurobindo gives a correspondent a vivid idea of the fundamental obstacles that oppose those who turn to Yoga. He is speaking of the discipline which is necessary when the soul, withdrawing its consent from the play of Nature, decides to put into practice the mastery which it has only

[1] *Katha Upanishad:* First cycle: Third Chapter: v. 14.

possessed so far in theory. "The psychic (being) has always been veiled," he writes, "consenting to the play of the mind, vital and physical (beings), experiencing everything through them in the ignorant vital, mental and physical way. How then can it be that they are bound to change at once when it just takes the trouble to whisper, 'Let there be Light'? They have a tremendous negating power and can refuse and do refuse point-blank. The mind resists with an obstinate persistency in argument and a constant confusion of ideas, the vital with a fury of bad will aided by the mind's obliging reasonings on its side, the physical resists with an obstinate inertia and crass fidelity to old habit, and when they have done, the general Nature comes in and says, 'What, you are going to get free from me so early? Not if I know it,' and it besieges and throws back the old nature on you again and again as long as it can."[1]

Human nature can never entirely get free from the pressure of the inconscience of the material world, from which it has arisen. Consciousness as it grows in the being has always had to struggle out of the Ignorance. "Human nature," Sri Aurobindo observes, "is made of that Ignorance and the character of the individual is made from the elements of the Ignorance. It is largely mechanistic like everything else in material Nature and there is almost invariably a resistance and, more often than not, a strong and stubborn resistance to any change demanded from it."[2]

Because the tamasic element is powerful in the physical nature the resistance there is very obstinate; it is full of inertia and has a constant tendency "to despond and despair, to give up, renounce the aim and the endeavour, collapse".[3] And though the sattwic element, by its turning

[1] *Letters*, Vol. II, p. 103.
[2] Ibid., Vol. I, p. 286.
[3] Ibid., p. 288.

towards the light, and the rajasic element by its desire for action and progress, can both be made to support the spiritual endeavour, they can also resist it. The sattwic ego is "the snare of virtue and self-righteousness, the ties of philanthropy, mental idealizations, family affections".[1] It frequently expresses itself in the compulsion to convert others to its own religious viewpoint and in that monopolistic attitude to the faith it serves as being the final and crowning revelation of God, which often characterizes the religious (as distinct from the spiritual) consciousness.[2] Nothing, Sri Aurobindo has observed somewhere, is so hard to shake as the fixed egoism of virtue. The sattwic element can also resist "by attachment to old ideas, to preconceived notions, to mental preferences and partial judgements, to opinions and reasonings which come in the way of higher truth and to which it is attached".[3] Most of us who have been brought up since childhood in a particular faith and with a knowledge of its dogmas and doctrines must experience this resistance of the sattwic

---

[1] *Letters*, Vol. II, p. 399.
[2] This distinction between the religious and the spiritual life is one we are not accustomed to make in the West. They are, says Sri Aurobindo, quite different and one must not confuse them. He characterizes them as follows: "The religious life is a movement of the ignorant human consciousness, turning or trying to turn away from the earth towards the Divine but as yet without knowledge and led by the dogmatic tenets and rules of some sect or creed which claims to have found the way out of the bonds of the earth-consciousness into some beatific Beyond. The religious life may be the first approach to the spiritual, but very often it is only a turning about in a round of rites, ceremonies and practices or set ideas and forms without any issue. The spiritual life, on the contrary, proceeds directly by a change of consciousness, a change from the ordinary consciousness, ignorant and separated from its true self and God, to a greater consciousness in which one finds one's true being and comes first into direct and living contact and then into union with the Divine. For the spiritual seeker this change of consciousness is the one thing he seeks and nothing else matters. . . . The spiritual life goes beyond the mind; it enters into the deeper consciousness of the Spirit and acts out of the truth of the Spirit." (*Letters*, Vol. I, pp. 90-1.)
[3] Ibid., p. 288.

ego, however deeply we may wish to become again as
plastic, open and receptive as "little children". Preconceptions can be a deadly obstacle in Yoga.

The obstructions of the rajasic element are in its
"desires and strong attachments, its vanity and self-
esteem, its constant habit of demand and many other
obstacles".[1] More difficult still is the violence and passion
brought to the aid of these by the vital resistance, for this,
says Sri Aurobindo, "is a source of all the acute difficulty,
revolt, upheavals and disorders which mar the course of
the yoga".[2] He goes on to explain: "The Divine is there,
but He does not ignore the conditions, the laws, the circumstances of Nature; it is under these conditions that He
does all His work in the world and man and consequently
in the sadhaka, the aspirant, even in the God-knower and
God-lover; even the saint and the sage continue to have
difficulties and to be limited by their human nature."[3]

As the unregenerate vital ego stands most in the way
of transformation, the vital difficulties that are liable to
afflict the aspirant are many and various. There is a part
of both the physical and vital nature which has not got
the will for *sadhana* and seeks any deprivation or dis-
appointment that may result from its discipline as an
excuse to overwhelm the *sadhaka* with doubt or depression. This vital condition produces the kind of reaction
which expresses itself in hopelessness, in revolt, despair
or a desire to leave the Yoga and abandon the spiritual
life. Temptation to give up the *sadhana* may also, of
course, be the result of the suggestions of hostile forces.

There are three extremely difficult obstacles to overcome in the vital being, Sri Aurobindo warns. These are
lust (sexual desire), wrath and rajasic ego. Against the
domination of these masterful impulses it is necessary to

[1] *Letters*, Vol II., p. 289.
[2] Ibid., p. 289.
[3] Ibid.

battle constantly, rejecting them with unflagging determination and a resolve to remain firm and undiscouraged, however persistent the attacks.

The mind and vital being are far more highly charged with egotism than the body, and it is the predilections of this 'I' of the self-regarding ego in all its sattwic, rajasic and tamasic elements, rooted into the nature and camouflaging itself with many subtle disguises, that so variously and persistently deflects and thwarts us. For egoism is in everyone. "Human nature," comments Sri Aurobindo, "is shot through in all its stuff with the thread of the ego; even when one tries to get away from it, it is in front or could be behind all the thoughts and actions like a shadow."[1]

To get rid of egoism is as difficult as making an entire surrender. Its disappearance means complete liberation.

The danger that, when the ordinary limits of the nature are broken down and a greater consciousness takes their place, a magnification of the ego may follow, is one of the great perils of the *sadhana* and to be watchfully and scrupulously guarded against. No one who is in the least human can avoid a thrill of delight and exaltation at this opening out of consciousness and its resultant experiences, nor should they: to cherish experiences, to be glad and humbly grateful for them, is a necessity constantly urged by Sri Aurobindo; what he desires the *sadhaka* to avoid is any puffing up of the ego, or if he cannot altogether avoid it, to watch it carefully and reject it.

Fluctuations in the force of the aspiration and the power of the *sadhana* may also create difficulty, but this is common to all aspirants and unavoidable. Lulls or arrests always occur: "One might almost say," Sri Aurobindo remarks, "that every step forward is followed by an arrest—at least, that is a very common, if not a universal experience."[2]

[1] *Letters*, Vol. II, pp. 425-6.
[2] *Letters*, Vol. IV, p. 277.

Many people find the conflict which springs up between their higher and lower consciousness very disturbing, first one and then the other in control and each continually struggling for mastery. But this separation of consciousness, as we saw in the chapter on 'The Luminous Crypt of the Soul', is necessary and good, so long as we do not attempt to condone or encourage the lower nature in any way.

To a disciple who was upset by the compulsion to speak and act in a way that he knew to be wrong, he wrote: "Even the experience which so alarms you, of states of consciousness in which you say and do things contrary to your true will, is not a reason for despair. It is a common experience in one form or another of all who try to rise above their ordinary nature. Not only those who practise Yoga, but religious men and those who seek only a moral control and self-improvement are confronted with this difficulty. . . . It is the lower elements which are being made to revolt consciously against the higher will. There then seems to be for a time a division in the nature, because the true being and all that supports it stand back and separate from these lower elements. At one time the true being occupies the field of the nature, at another the lower nature used by some contrary Force pushes it back and seizes the ground—and this we now see while formerly the thing happened but the nature of the happening was not clear to us. If there is a firm will to progress, this division is overpassed."[1]

The sinking down of the consciousness as the result of fatigue, of some adverse touch or wrong movement; the comparative rapidity with which the radiance of an experience may be swallowed up; the cessation of experiences; the sense of desertion or sterility; disturbances to the nervous system or body by the pressure of vital

[1] *Letters*, Vol. IV, pp. 283-4.

difficulties or the inertia of the physical being which changes very slowly and often cannot keep up with the changes on higher levels: all these things may afflict the seeker.

A long continuity of higher experiences can produce in the physical mind "a sense of exhaustion or reaction of unease or dullness".[1] The power to relax; to sleep enough and to eat sensibly if the body and nervous system are overtaxed; the refuge of some interesting work to do as a support if suffering a check or temporary reverse, are all things that can be made to assist the aspirant through difficult phases.

These alternations of light and darkness, as of joy and trouble in ordinary life, are not a proof of incapacity or predestined failure, Sri Aurobindo comments, but the result of the nature of human consciousness. "One has to be prepared for them and pass through."[2]

As well as these more common difficulties that affect everyone there are also dangers. "If you aim high," Sri Aurobindo writes, "there is always the danger of a steep fall if you misconduct your aeroplane. But the danger is for those who allow themselves to entertain a double

[1] *Bases of Yoga*, p. 47.
[2] *Letters*, Vol. II, p. 339. Certain very stubborn difficulties may be encountered when the aspirant descends in the course of the *sadhana* from the mental or the higher vital plane to the physical consciousness. The higher levels may be sustained by "plenty of vigour and verve and interest", but the descent to conquer "the physical bedrock", as Sri Aurobindo calls it, is always "accompanied by a fading of the first deep experiences and a descent to the neutral obscure inertia which is the bedrock of the unredeemed physical nature. It is there that the Light, the Power, the Ananda of the Divine has to descend and transform everything, driving away for ever all obscurity and all inertia. . . . It is a period when doubt, denial, dryness, greyness and all kindred things come up with a great force and often reign completely for a time. It is after this stage has been successfully crossed that the true light begins to come, the light which is not of the mind but of the spirit." (Ibid., p. 445 passim.)

being,[1] aiming high but also indulging their lower outlook and hankerings. What else can you expect when people do that? You must become single-minded, then the difficulties of the mind and vital (being) will be overcome."[2] To imagine that a high stage of advancement in Yoga automatically protects the aspirant from running into disaster is a total misapprehension. The higher the development the more scrupulous must be the care, for to fall from a great height is much likelier to prove fatal.[3]

The dangers presented by entry into the intermediate zones, such as the vital world, which may attend an extension of consciousness, need also to be kept in mind. In *The Life Divine* Sri Aurobindo speaks of the "chaos of unfamiliar and supernormal experiences . . . (the) press of subliminal or cosmic forces, subconscient mental, vital, subtle-physical" which may engulf the aspirant before "the tranquillizing purification of the outer nature has been affected"[4] should he, by one means or another, break

---

[1] The duality in human nature—the "two Personae, one bright one dark" that is in every human being—is something from which nobody can escape, Sri Aurobindo writes. "If that were not there, Yoga would be an easy walk-over and there would be no struggle." Again he observes: "Every man is full of these contradictions, because he is one person, no doubt, but made up of different personalities. . . . So long as one does not aim at unity in a single dominant intention, like that of seeking and self-dedication to the Divine, they get on somehow together, alternating or quarrelling or muddling through or else one taking the lead and compelling the others to take a minor part—but once you try to unite them in one aim, then the trouble becomes evident." (*Letters*, Vol. II, pp. 345 and 354.)

[2] Ibid., p. 346.

[3] "The more intense the experiences that come, the higher the forces that descend, the greater become the possibilities of deviation and error. For the very intensity and the very height of the force excites and aggrandizes the movements of the lower nature and raises up in it all opposing elements in their full force, but often in the disguise of truth, wearing a mask of plausible justification. There is needed a great patience, calm, sobriety, balance, an impersonal detachment and sincerity free from all taint of ego or personal human desire." Ibid., p. 30.)

[4] *The Life Divine*, Vol. II (2), p. 932.

down the wall between the inner being and his outer awareness.

This occurrence may "unduly sway or chaotically drive the being, encircle it in a cave of darkness, or keep it wandering in a wilderness of glamour, allurement, deception, or push it into an obscure battlefield full of secret and treacherous and misleading or open and violent oppositions; beings and voices and influences may appear to the inner sense and vision and hearing claiming to be the Divine Being or His messengers or Powers and Godheads of the Light or guides of the path to realization, while in truth they are of a very different character".[1]

The perils of what another great Master has called this "astral glamour" are likely to ensnare any who are too egotistical, ambitious or vain; who are obscure in mind, vacillating in will, or absorbed by a strong passion; who suffer from a weakness, unsteadiness or want of balance of the life-force.

These dangers have always been known to spiritual experience. In the West it led mystics like St. John of the Cross to teach an entire rejection of what in modern parlance we should designate 'psychic' experience, while in the East, Sri Aurobindo remarks, they were met "by imposing the necessity of initiation, of discipline, of methods of purification and testing by ordeal, of an entire submission to the directions of . . . one who has realized the Truth and himself possesses and is able to communicate the light"; in short, the Master, Teacher, *Guru*. Nevertheless, he adds, the dangers can only be surmounted "if there is or there grows up a complete sincerity, a will for purity, a readiness to lose or subject to a divine yoke the limiting and self-affirming ego".[2]

Many people tread the path without being exposed on a major scale to these dangers; but nearly everyone ex-

[1] *The Life Divine*, Vol. II (2), p. 933.
[2] Ibid., pp. 933-4.

periences them in a small way. The subtle vital world (with which creative people are often in close touch) has an aspect of enchanting beauty, as may be seen in Coleridge's *Kubla Khan*; but its reverse side is full of horrible things and is responsible for much that is cruel, brutal and repulsive in human nature. Nightmares are contacts with this unpleasant world.[1]

The difficulties that rise from the obstacles in human nature itself are often complicated by—and perhaps are inseparable from—the interference of adverse forces which exist to obstruct the development of a higher consciousness in the world and are swift to exploit any weakness or wrong movement in the *sadhaka* in order to prevent his escape from the conditions of the Ignorance.

The psychology on which Yoga is based emphasizes the power of the element of free choice in human experience by the concept of *karma* (action-reaction); but it also makes clear that the ordinary individual is continually the focus of vast cosmic forces which determine him far more than he determines himself for great ages of his pilgrimage. The notion that all things rise from within is soon qualified in the practice of Yoga by the experience that, on the contrary, many things other than sense perceptions arrive from outside, enter by our own unconscious sanction and,

---

[1] To the problem of how the aspirant is to distinguish good from bad forces in Yoga, Sri Aurobindo has this to say: "Everything depends on the nature of the force and its working: what does it do, what seems to be its purpose? If it works to purify or open the system, or brings with it light or peace, or prepares the change of the thought, ideas, feelings, character in the sense of a turning towards a higher consciousness, then it is the right force. If it is dark or obscure or perturbs the being with rajasic or egoistic suggestions or excites the lower nature, then it is an adverse force." (*More Lights on Yoga*, p. 98.) Again: "To say that all light is good is as if you said that all water is good—or even that all clear or transparent water is good: it would not be true. . . . False lights exist and misleading lustres . . . One must therefore be on one's guard and distinguish; the true discrimination has to come by growth of the psychic feeling and a purified mind and experience. (*Bases of Yoga*, p. 63.)

because we do not recognize them until they have obtained possession of some part of our being, give us the illusion that they originated within.

All the ordinary vital movements are foreign to the true being and come from outside, Sri Aurobindo states: "they do not belong to the soul nor do they originate in it but are waves from the general Nature, Prakriti."

The desires come from outside, enter the subconscious vital (being) and rise to the surface. It is only when they rise to the surface and the mind becomes aware of them that we become conscious of the desire. It seems to be our own because we feel it thus rising from the vital (being) into the mind and do not know that it came from outside. What belongs to the vital (nature), to the being, what makes it responsible is not the desire itself, but the habit of responding to the waves or the currents of suggestion that come into it from the universal Prakriti."[1]

In another place he comments: "Our nature is a constant activity of forces supplied to us out of which (or rather out of a small amount of it) we make what we will or can. What we make seems fixed and formed for good, but in reality all is a play of forces, a flux, nothing fixed or stable; the appearance or stability is given by constant repetition and recurrence of the same vibrations and formations."[2]

II

THE CAUSES OF DIFFICULTY

THE path need not be cut by periodical violent storms, Sri Aurobindo observes, though the fact that it is so disturbed for a great many people is obvious: but provided the aspirant sticks to it, after a certain point these

[1] *The Bases of Yoga*, p. 72.
[2] Ibid., pp. 106-7.

storms diminish in frequency and force. Different temperaments naturally react variously to the difficulties of Yoga; for some there are sharp ups and downs, sailings on top of the wave only to plunge into the trough; for others the course is serene, not because they do not have difficulties to overcome, but because they are perfectly confident of the Divine Presence supporting them continually.

A blind acquiescence to ordeal, however, or any cult of suffering for its own sake in the pietistic belief that it is sent by God, is no part of Integral Yoga. A firm and therefore positive will and a clear intelligence in the mind are inestimably valuable to the *sadhak* and Sri Aurobindo is always at pains to explain to his disciples the causes that lie behind their troubles, so that they may understand them, and, putting themselves actively on the side of the Divine, who is working all the time to eliminate the impurities, may co-operate with Him in the task of transformation.

Those who like thorns in the flesh will probably keep them, but those who see that mental suffering, like bodily illness, is a sign of disharmony, will realize that the first thing demanded of them is to remove its causes and utterly cast them out, not to embrace it as something virtuous in itself.

The unpleasant emulation of suffering that has marred a great deal of Western mysticism—it would seem to have reached its extreme in mystics like Suso—has tended to maroon itself in the dark night of Good Friday and to ignore that Jesus' beatitude lay in the final triumph of Easter Day. It may be a grave presumption in us to imagine that the suffering voluntarily accepted by the Avatar, not out of his *imperfection* but out of his *perfection*, as the price of his descent into the conditions of this world, necessarily assumes a divine nature in anyone else.

"All undelight, all pain and suffering," Sri Aurobindo writes, "are a sign of imperfection, of incompleteness; they arise from a division of being, an incompleteness of consciousness of being, an incompleteness of the force of being."[1] Elsewhere he remarks that the vital being has a tendency to cling to suffering, because it likes the drama of it, and that it is a dangerous trait in human nature, to be firmly expelled by all who practise Yoga.

The central difficulty of the *sadhana* is that of attuning the nature with the working of the Divine Light and Power. If the aspirant can get this solved, Sri Aurobindo states, the other difficulties will either disappear or take a subordinate place. If we realize clearly enough the greatness of the undertaking involved in Yoga, we shall avoid much unnecessary despondency and not feel sunk in gloom when, after what seems a long endeavour, we find we are not on the mountain-top but just approaching the foothills.

What causes lie most persistently behind the dry periods in Yoga? As Sri Aurobindo has already explained, the unwillingness of the outer nature to give up its sovereignty and submit to a higher leadership is one of the principal stumbling-blocks. Our desire for transformation, however deep and sincere in our inner being, cannot change in a flash the nature that we have built up so laboriously and accepted in all its limitations for an untold succession of life-experiences. Many of the most obstinate *samskaras*[2] we have to cope with in ourselves come from the deep past that lies behind us. "We bring most of ourselves—or rather most of our predispositions, tendencies of reaction to the universal Nature, from past lives. Heredity only affects strongly the external being; besides all the effects of heredity are not accepted even there, only

[1] *The Life Divine*, Vol. II (2), p. 1116.
[2] *Samskaras*: Fixed mental formations; impressions of past habits; experiences stored up in the subconscious. (*More Lights on Yoga*, p. 139.)

those that are in consonance with what we are to be or
not preventive of it at least."[1]

In ordinary life the vital movements of anger, greed,
sex, desire, are accepted as natural and legitimate unless
they become anti-social in their manifestation. In the
spiritual life the complete conquest of these things is demanded. "That is why the struggle is more felt," Sri
Aurobindo observes, "not because these things rise more
strongly in sadhakas than in ordinary men, but because of
the intensity of the struggle between the spiritual mind
which demands control and the vital movements which
rebel and want to continue in the new as they did in the
old life."

He goes on to say that there are many things in the
ordinary man of which he is not conscious "because the
vital hides them from the mind and gratifies them without
the mind realizing what is the force that is moving the
action—thus things that are done under the plea of altru-
ism, philanthropy, service, etc., are largely moved by the
ego which hides itself behind these justifications. In Yoga
the secret motive has to be pulled out from behind the
veil, exposed and got rid of. Secondly, some things are
suppressed and not eliminated; they may rise up any day
or they may express themselves in various nervous forms
or other disorders of the mind or vital (being) or body
without it being evident what is their real cause. . . . Here
again, in sadhana one has to become conscious of these
suppressed impulses and eliminate them."[2]

All this requires a candour and sincerity very difficult
to human nature. It can only be achieved by spiritual
endeavour and needs "a severity of introspective self-
vision, an unsparing scrutiny of self-observation of which
many sadhakas and even Yogis are not capable and it is
only by an illuminating Grace that reveals the sadhaka to

1 *Bases of Yoga*, p. 108.
2 *Letters*, Vol. I, 296 passim.

himself and transforms what is deficient in him that it can
be done. And then only if he himself consents and lends
himself wholly to the divine working."[1]

There is another cause of difficulty. In the same way
that the human body cannot stand too much sunlight
without gradual adaptation to it, so the human consciousness cannot at first bear or absorb a constant descent of
the Divine Light or Bliss or Force. It needs, says Sri
Aurobindo, periods of assimilation: "but this assimilation
goes on behind the veil of the surface consciousness, the
experience or the realization that has descended retires
behind the veil and leaves this outer or surface consciousness to lie fallow and become ready for a new descent. In
the more developed stages of the Yoga these dark or dull
periods become shorter, less trying as well as uplifted by
the sense of a greater consciousness which, though not
acting for immediate progress, yet remains and sustains
the outer nature."[2]

A further cause of dullness is a resistance in the nature,
either from some element in it which is not ready or is
unwilling to change, or which has not felt any descent
there may have been. This resistance may come from "a
strong habitual formation of the mind or the vital (being)
or some temporary inertia of the physical consciousness and not exactly a part of the nature—and this,
whether showing or concealing itself, thrusts up the
obstacle."[3]

These periods of preparation and assimilation are
universal. They should be accepted patiently and without
resentment. The acting Force has to lift up part of the
nature on to a higher level and then come down to a lower
level to raise that up too, and this movement of ascent
and descent is often "extremely trying" because of the

[1] *Letters*, Vol. I, p. 299.
[2] *Bases of Yoga*, pp. 54-5.
[3] Ibid., p. 55.

inability of the mind and vital being "to understand or follow the intricate movement".¹

Nevertheless the transforming Force knows better than "our mental ignorance or our vital impatience" what is required in this complicated process of purification and growth. Unless the imperfections latent or active in the being are raised up into the light where they can be seen and combated, how can they be eradicated? No one can struggle to change what he does not know; therefore those who, through Yoga, commit themselves to the Light, must not feel daunted when the darkness also leaps into being under its impact.

As we have already mentioned, the things that create the difficulties in Yoga are not simply internal but also external. There are forces of the cosmic Ignorance which cannot be exhausted. In time their attacks may lose strength and diminish, but only if the soul rejects them, aided by the Divine, each time they make an assault.

The hostile forces are in the world to maintain the Ignorance. They lay siege and may make a mass attack to overpower, using any weakness they can find and exploit in the aspirant in order to breach his defences, for this is the *point d'appui* without which they would be powerless. But at each resistance a 'hedgehog' is won against them and a new part of the being secured to the Light.

The attacks of these cosmic forces, Sri Aurobindo comments, commonly become violent when the progress is growing rapid or definite. Any approach by the *sadhaka* to "the gates of the Kingdom of Light . . . makes these forces rage and they strain every nerve and use or create every opportunity to turn the sadhak back or, if possible, drive him out of the path altogether by their suggestions, their violent influences and their exploitation of all kinds of incidents that always crop up more and more when

¹ *Bases of Yoga*, p. 59.

these conditions prevail, so that he may not reach the gates".[1]

Yet these hostile forces,[2] he reminds us, possess a certain self-chosen function; "it is to test the condition of the individual, of the work, of the earth itself and their readiness for the spiritual descent and fulfilment".[3] Therefore they are present at each step to discourage, criticize, incite to revolt, doubt, unbelief and in every possible way to amass difficulties.

The existence of these forces and their destructive influence should be given a healthy regard but not allowed to become an easy way of escaping responsibility. It is very soothing and comforting to be able to heap one's troubles on to an external agent, rather than upon one's own imperfections, but it is precisely this kind of ostrich-attitude which creates its own formidable difficulty in *sadhana*.

These two great sources of trouble in Yoga, the resistances within the individual's own nature and the resistance of the universal Nature[4] which does not wish the being to escape from its bondage into the light, may induce a pressure of conditions that cause mental and vital suffering.[5] There is, however, no invariable rule of such suffer-

[1] *Letters*, Vol. II, p. 450.
[2] "The hostile forces are anti-divine, not merely undivine; they make use of the lower nature, pervert it, fill it with distorted movements and by that means influence man and even try to enter and possess or at least entirely control him." (*Bases of Yoga*, p. 50.)
[3] Ibid., p. 66.
[4] "This may take the form of a vehement insistence in the continuation of the old movements, waves of them thrown on the mind and vital (being) and body so that old ideas, impulses, desires, feelings, responses continue even after they are thrown out and rejected, and can return like an invading army from outside, until the whole nature, given to the Divine, refuses to admit them." (*Letters*, Vol. I, p. 285.)
[5] "Those who fall, fall not because of the attacks of the vital forces, but because they put themselves on the side of the hostile Forces and prefer a vital ambition or desire (ambition, vanity, lust, etc.) to the spiritual *siddhi*." (*Letters*, Vol. II, p. 489.)

ing. Far from being the badge of sanctity, it is the mark of interior tension and divided being and it remains as long as these conditions continue.

We may mistakenly imagine that it is the soul in us that suffers and secretly hope that there is a saving element of nobility in the more searching of our pains: but the soul does not suffer. "The Self" Sri Aurobindo observes, "is calm and equal to all things and the only sorrow of the psychic being is the sorrow of the resistance of Nature to the Divine Will. . . . What is affected by suffering is the vital nature and the body."[1]

III

THE RIGHT ATTITUDE IN DIFFICULTY

THE secret of the right attitude to take in difficulty is contained in Sri Aurobindo's description of his system of spiritual practice as 'a sunlit way'. It is the secret of an absolute trust in the Divine; of a quiet and happy confidence and faith in the aspirant's own divine potentialities, whatever obstacles lie in the course of their unfoldment; and of a steady affirmation of all that the positive way enjoins.

In order to understand this better, let us look for a moment at some of the things Sri Aurobindo has written about the distinctive characteristics of the sunlit path and the qualities which it requires in those who chose it.

As we have already seen, Sri Aurobindo, though he does not in any way condemn the negative means for those who wish to get away from life, states that they are disadvantageous from the positive point of view and the attempt to transform life. In another context, defining the negative and positive means of removing difficulties, he

[1] *Letters*, Vol. I, p. 284.

explains: "By negative I mean merely repressing the desires and wrong movements and egoism, by positive I mean the bringing down of light and peace and purity in those parts from above. I do not mean that these movements are not to be rejected—but all the energy should not be used solely for rejection. It must also be directed to the positive replacement of them by the higher consciousness. The more this consciousness comes, the easier also will the rejection be."[1]

Contrasting the Dark and the Sunlit Paths—the negative and affirmative ways—he writes: "The dark path is there and there are many who make, like the Christians, a Gospel of spiritual suffering; many hold it to be so under certain circumstances, as it has been in so many lives at the beginning, or one may choose to make it so. But then the price has to be paid with resignation, fortitude or a tenacious resilience. I admit that, if borne in that way, the attacks of the dark forces or the ordeals they impose have a meaning. After each victory gained over them, there is then a sensible advance; often they seem to show us the difficulties in ourselves which we have to overcome and to say: 'Here you must conquer'; all the same it is a too dark and difficult way which nobody should follow on whom the necessity does not lie."[2]

In another place, speaking of the practice of *vairāgya* (turning away from life), he admits its occasional utility as a counterbalance to a too strong vital pull, but says that it tends, through a *tamasic* element of despair and depression, to "dilapidate the fire of the being and may lead in some cases to falling between two stools so that one loses earth and misses heaven".[3]

He therefore prefers to replace *vairagya* by a quiet,

[1] *Letters*, Vol. IV, pp. 365-6.
[2] *Letters*, Vol. I, pp. 302-3.
[3] *Letters*, Vol. IV, pp. 395.

resolute rejection of wrong movements. This rejection does not include the destruction of any of those activities and powers, such as painting, music, poetry, which can be made instruments of the Yoga and the divine work, but these must find a new and spiritual base. "Yoga can be done without the rejection of life," he writes, "without killing or impairing the life-joy or the vital force."[1] Any inclination to deny life or the world and disappear into the Indefinable he objects to *as being incompatible with this Yoga*, with its aim of bringing the Divine into life.

There are certain conditions necessary for following the sunlit path, principally that the psychic being is constantly or usually in front, or that there is a natural spirit of surrender and faith or a face turned habitually to the sun. If the psychic being is strong and master of the being there is little or no subjective suffering. Instead "the way is sunlit and a great joy and sweetness are the note of the whole sadhana".[2]

Sri Aurobindo teaches that true vision rises above what he calls the "intellectual-ethical virtue-and-sin dodge which is only a mental construction of practical value for the outward life but not a truth of inner values"[3] and sees only harmonies and disharmonies which must be set right. Obstacles, he says, "have to be looked at as something wrong in the machinery of human nature which has to be changed—they should not be regarded as sins or wrong-doings which make one despair of oneself and the sadhana".[4]

A seeing of ourselves and of all the complex forces that move on the stage of our being, not from any dry outer intellectual or ethical viewpoint, but from an inner spiritual observation, "a living perception of how things

[1] *Letters*, Vol. II, p. 395.
[2] *Letters*, Vol. I. p. 286.
[3] *Letters*, Vol. II, p. 353.
[4] Ibid., p. 407.

are done in us", can be intensely interesting and bring "a living mastery over this inner universe".[1]

Wonderful indeed would be the aspirant who could escape, in the early stages of the sadhana, some periods in which he did not feel like a fly caught helplessly in the intricate web woven about him by his nature; nevertheless the habit of dispassion, urged by Sri Aurobindo, of quiet and detached interest in all the arduous and yet marvellous task of transformation which the Divine Master initiates in every being he calls to Yoga, can be the staunchest of supports in the sadhana.

The artist, struggling to create, possesses this power to be steadfastly centred in the processes of his task and to feel an absorbed interest even when the material seems to rebel, knowing that each solution found to the problems of his art brings him nearer greater mastery, and this is the attitude to the difficulties of Yoga which every sadhaka should possess.

Those aspirants who allow their faults or failures to depress or discourage them unduly, only make the way rougher.[2] "It does not matter what defects you may have in your nature," Sri Aurobindo says encouragingly. "The one thing that matters is keeping yourself open to the Force. Nobody can transform himself by his own unaided efforts; it is only the Divine Force that can transform him. If you keep yourself open, all the rest will be done for you."[3]

Despondency and shame, ideas of incapacity and a dwelling on defects are weakening things. One should not

---

[1] Letters, Vol. II, p. 352.

[2] "Imperfections, even many and serious imperfections, cannot be a permanent bar to progress in the Yoga. . . . If imperfections were a bar, then no man could succeed in Yoga; for all are imperfect, and I am not sure, from what I have seen, that it is not those who have the greatest power for Yoga who have very often, or have had, the greatest imperfections." (Bases of Yoga, p. 53.)

[3] Ibid., p. 30.

always be thinking of defects and wrong movements but concentrate primarily on what one is trying to be. "Turn your eyes more to the coming light," he tells a disciple, "and less to any immediate darkness."[1] To be constantly observing faults and failures causes depression and discourages the faith.

In another place he writes: "Free yourself from all exaggerated self-depreciation and the habit of getting depressed by the sense of sin, difficulty or failure. These feelings do not really help, on the contrary, they are an immense obstacle and hamper the progress. They belong to the religious, not to the Yogic mentality."[2] The *sadhaka* must look on all defects as movements of the lower nature, common to all, and reject them, "calmly, firmly and persistently with full confidence in the Divine Power—without weakness or depression or negligence and without excitement, impatience or violence".[3]

Too continual an emphasis on the dark side of things only increases the force of the difficulties. "It is a subtle law of the action of consciousness that if you stress difficulties—you have to observe them, of course, but not stress them, they will quite sufficiently do that for themselves—the difficulties tend to stick or even increase; on the contrary if you put your whole stress on faith and aspiration and concentrate steadily on what you aspire to, that will sooner or later tend towards realization."[4] This

---

[1] *Bases of Yoga*, p. 49.
[2] Ibid., pp. 50-1.
[3] Ibid.
[4] *Letters*, Vol. I, p. 309. Those who are easily discouraged may be reassured to know that Sri Aurobindo himself said that in his own case Yoga had always been 'a battle'. "It took me four years of inner striving to find a real way, even though the divine help was with me all the time, and even then, it seemed to come by an accident; and it took me ten years more of intense yoga under a supreme inner guidance to trace it out and that was because I had my past and the world's past to assimilate and overpass before I could find and found the future." (*Letters*, Vol. II, pp. 389-90.)

mood of affirmation was well stressed in the injunction: *Whatsoever things ye desire when ye pray, believe that ye have received them and ye shall have them.*

Always fight out the difficulty at once, says Sri Aurobindo, and hold on resolutely to the idea that, taken in the right attitude, adversity becomes an opportunity for advance. And the only right attitude is to become always more quiet, firmer in the will to go through to the end; to open more and more effectually to the Light; to continue to make "an affirmation of faith even in the midst of obscurity, faith in the presence of a Power that is working behind the cloud and the veil, in the guidance of the Guru, by an observation of oneself to find any cause of the arrest, not in a spirit of depression or discouragement but with the will to find out and remove it".[1]

A quiet, steady rejection of defects, made in absolute sincerity (the *sine qua non* of the Yoga) will finally cast them out, for, as Sri Aurobindo observes, each victory means new strength for further victories.

To indulge a desire or false movement will often give a worse recoil in the *sadhana* than to disappoint it, and in the later stages to give in over a small point may mean losing a whole battle, so important do even minor details become. If the vital or mental being are exposed to disturbing touches, the answer is to live more deeply within, for the inmost psychic being "is not oppressed by them; it stands in its own closeness to the Divine and sees the small surface movements as surface things foreign to the true Being".[2]

There are always difficulties in the beginning for all aspirants; even for the advanced, the Vedic sages tell us, there are still problems: "As one ascends from peak to peak, there is made clear the much that has still to be done." Therefore in the beginning of your practice, Sri

[1] *Letters*, Vol. IV, p. 377.
[2] *Bases of Yoga*, p. 51.

Aurobindo says, be patient; a slow development is the best anyone can hope for in the first years. Cherish the small beginnings. The Yogin knows "that the neutral quiet[1] so dissatisfying to the vital eagerness of the sadhaka is the first step towards the peace that passeth all understanding, the small current or thrill of inner delight the first trickling of the ocean of Ananda, the play of lights or colours, the key of the doors of the inner vision and experience, the descent that stiffens the body into a concentrated stillness the first touch of something at the end of which is the presence of the Divine. He is not impatient; he is rather careful not to disturb the evolution that is beginning."[2] Moderation, he cautions, is needed even in the eagerness for progress. "People who are cheerful and ready to go even slowly step by step, march faster and more securely than those who are impatient and in haste."[3]

Depression is a negative thing, like fear, and belongs to the vital. It is "a clouded grey state" which obstructs the inner light and increases difficulty, and he quotes the injunction of the *Gita*: "Yoga should be practised persistently with a heart free from depression."[4]

A constant recurrence of despair, despondency, doubt and revolt are often due to mental or vital formations which seize the vital mind at the slightest excuse and make it revolve in the same well-worn circle, in the same mechanical way that the body responds to the habit of illness. Make the vital mind once withdraw its consent

[1] "It was on what you call emptiness," Sri Aurobindo wrote to a disciple, "that my whole Yoga was founded and it was through it that there came afterwards all the inexhaustible riches of a greater knowledge, will and joy, all the experiences of a greater mental, psychic and vital realm, all the ranges up to Overmind and beyond. The cup has often to be emptied before it can be new-filled, the Yogin, the sadhak ought not to be afraid of emptiness or silence." (*Letters*, Vol. I, p. 389.)
[2] Ibid., pp. 319-20.
[3] Ibid., pp. 317-18.
[4] Ibid., p. 304.

from these habitual movements and refuse to believe in
the suggestions or feelings that start them and they will
cease. A firm pressure of expulsion is always a better way
to deal with resistances or hostile suggestions than to
struggle with them, for all reactions that disturb the
quietude and cover up the inner being, mitigate against
an easy outcome. The most important thing is to become
quieter and quieter, Sri Aurobindo says; to look on an
adverse influence as something which has intruded; to
separate yourself from it, deny it, and abide in a quiet
confidence in the Divine Power.

   This quiet confidence is to be distinguished from self-
assurance, as true humility is to be distinguished from that
self-depreciation that expresses itself in an ostentatious
parade of being sinful, which is the negative inversion of
spiritual pride. Nevertheless, because Sri Aurobindo
always comes down firmly on the use of the positive
qualities in the *sadhana*, he maintains that an excessive
optimism is better and more helpful in *sadhana* than an
excessive pessimism.

   This does not mean sailing blithely along without
noticing one's faults. To recognize wrong movements[1] of
idea, feeling, speech or action is the first condition of inner
progress. It means learning that equanimity which is not
touched or troubled by anything said or done to one,
seeing them "with a straight look, free from the distortions
created by personal feeling, and to try to understand what
is behind them, why they happen, what is to be learnt
from them, what is it in oneself which they are cast against
and what inner profit or progress one can make out of
them; it means self-mastery over the vital movements—
anger and sensitiveness and pride as well as desire and the
rest—not to let them get hold of the emotional being and

   [1] "By wrong is meant what departs from the truth, from the higher
consciousness and higher self, from the way of the Divine." (*Letters*,
Vol. I, p. 326.)

disturb the inner peace, not to speak and act in the rush and impulsion of these things, always to act and speak out of a calm inner poise of the spirit. . . . Equality means another thing—to have an equal view of men and their nature and acts and the forces that move them; it helps one to see truth about them by pushing away from the mind all personal feelings in one's seeing and judgement and even all the mental bias."[1] This equanimity is certainly not easy, but one should always try to make it increasingly the basis of one's inner state and outer movements.

Just as there are forces concerned to depress and discourage, so there are also forces to restore and strengthen, and the aspirant must develop the power to draw upon these resources. Once something of the Truth has shown within "it will always, even if for a time heavily clouded over with wrong movements, shine out again like the sun in heaven. Therefore persevere with confidence and never lose courage."[2]

There is strength even in the weakest. No formation of strength or weakness is final; at any moment it may change, and does so change, we are told, particularly under the pressure of Yoga, where at any moment there may be seen "weakness changing into power, the incapable becoming capable, suddenly or slowly the instrumental consciousness rising to a new stature or developing its latent powers".[3] Spiritual endeavour does not depend for its success on the determined will of the aspirant; it depends on a combination of his will with the help given by the Divine Power.

---

[1] *Letters*, Vol. I, pp. 324-5. "When there is an attack from the human instruments of adverse forces, one should try to overcome it not in a spirit of personal hatred or anger or wounded egoism, but with a calm spirit of strength and equanimity and a call to the Divine Force to act. Success or failure lies with the Divine." (*Letters*, Vol. IV, p. 376.)

[2] *Letters*, Vol. IV, p. 408.

[3] Ibid., p. 394.

Dryness in Yoga can be greatly reduced, as has been stressed already, if the *sadhaka* has what Sri Aurobindo calls an ardour of introspection and self-conquest and finds every step of the effort and struggle interesting. It is also reduced if the aspirant can once achieve that trust which feels the hand of the Divine in each turn of the path, and the grace and guidance even in difficulty, but at the same time does not always demand or expect to understand its workings.

The secret of weathering the ordeals of the path, as in so much else in the Yoga, lies in the heart, not in the mind, though the mind, by holding firmly to the truth in attacks, can by its alliance greatly assist, especially in those stages before the psychic being has fully come forward. If the psychic being is to the fore, difficulties are not felt as definitive but as imperfections which the Grace will remove: once the heart can open its inner doors "the soul looks out in a blaze of trust and self-giving. Before that fire the debates of the mind and its difficulties wither away and the path however long or arduous becomes a sunlit road not only towards but through love and Ananda."[1]

Few can attain such rightfulness of spirit at first, but patient constancy will win it. "Grumble," says Sri Aurobindo to a disciple in difficulties, "if your nature compels you to it, but persevere,"[2] and his final word to all those experiencing trouble is contained in the simple instruction: "Be faithful and you will conquer."[3]

[1] *Letters*, Vol. I, p. 294.
[2] Ibid., p. 295.
[3] *Letters, Bases of Yoga, Lights on Yoga, More Lights on Yoga, The Yoga and its Objects*, passim.

CHAPTER VI

SADHANA IN ORDINARY LIFE

This is an exceedingly difficult aim and difficult Yoga; to many or most it will seem impossible. All the established forces of the ordinary ignorant world-consciousness are opposed to it and deny it and try to prevent it, and the sadhak will find his own mind, life and body full of the most obstinate impediments to its realization. If you can accept the ideal whole-heartedly, face all the difficulties, leave the past and its ties behind you and are ready to give up everything and risk everything for this divine possibility, then only can you hope to discover by experience the Truth behind it. *Lights on Yoga*, p. 1.

One must not enter on this path, far vaster and more arduous than most ways of Yoga, unless one is sure of the psychic call and of one's readiness to go through to the end. Ibid., p. 3.

Yoga is directed towards God, not towards man. If a divine supramental consciousness and power can be brought down and established in the material world, that obviously would mean an immense change for the earth including humanity and its life. But the effect on humanity would only be one result of the change; it cannot be the object of the sadhana. The object of the sadhana can only be to live in the divine consciousness and to manifest it in life. *Letters*, Vol. I, p. 87.

SRI AUROBINDO was often asked whether it was possible to practise *sadhana* in 'worldly' or ordinary life, as distinct from practising it in his Ashram, and he laid down certain conditions and gave a number of recommendations concerning this question.

The distinction between *sadhana* in ordinary life and *sadhana* in the Ashram is not such a radical one as it might appear, as can be seen by the following statements of Sri Aurobindo on the nature of his Ashram: "This Ashram," he writes, "has been created with another

144

object than that ordinarily common to such institutions, not for the renunciation of the world but as a centre and a field of practice for the evolution of another kind and form of life which would in the final end be moved by a higher spiritual consciousness and embody a greater life of the spirit."[1] And again: "This is not an Ashram like others—the members are not Sannyasis (ascetics); it is not *moksha* (liberation) that is the sole aim of the Yoga here."[2]

To those living in the West who have at present no choice other than that of practising Yoga in ordinary life, Sri Aurobindo's opinions on the subject are naturally of importance. The advantages are certainly not to be minimized of living in a community where everyone is concentrated upon the same aim, under the guidance of a Teacher and in an atmosphere obviously extremely helpful in every way. If the pressure is greater, so is the help and force that are available, nearer and more intense.

But there are disadvantages as well as advantages to every way of life. The aspirant doing Yoga in ordinary life, in having to stand on his own feet and not only accept the material insecurities and challenges of existence, which are lifted from the inmate of a spiritual institution, but also the inner difficulties common to them both, has no cause to fear that he is not facing life and its trials firmly or that he is shirking his adult responsibilities.[3]

---

[1] *Letters*, Vol. II, p. 465. [2] Ibid., p. 470.

[3] The type of extreme ascetism exemplified for the West by the Enclosed Orders would seem to be no longer envisaged as desirable in this age by the most modern teachings coming from the East. Ramana Maharshi appears always to have discouraged the renouncement of home and property, saying "true renunciation is the renunciation of desires, passions and attachments". (See *Ramana Maharshi and the Path of Self-Knowledge*, p. 72.) Sri Aurobindo considered anyone who thought in terms of 'renouncement' unready for Integral Yoga, since the aspirant must be convinced the world is "ugly, stupid, brutal and full of intolerable suffering" as a precondition. (*More Lights on Yoga*, p. 69.) The Buddhist point of view on this subject is interestingly debated by J. Evola in *The Doctrine of Awakening*, pp. 128–30. See also *The Heart of Buddhist Meditation*, by Nyanaponika Thera, pp. 116, 120–1.

On the other hand the ordinary life of the world is in many ways inimical to spiritual change. At every attempt to consolidate his growth into a higher consciousness, the aspirant has nearly always to encounter an intense counter-pull from those about him who do not wish for change, who are content with the ordinary life and consciousness, or worse still, are often alarmed at the prospect that he is changing at all and do their best consciously or unconsciously to prevent it.

He also bears on his shoulders the full weight of responsibility for the practical application of the *sadhana* in his life and must be in every way his own disciplinarian. Because he is, inwardly at all events, a solitary, he must interpret the teaching even more impartially, be even more scrupulous, vigilant, discriminating and remorsely honest than those who have someone directly in authority over them to correct, check, help and support them.

Answering a query as to whether a certain individual should enter the Ashram or remain among family duties, Sri Aurobindo said: "The question about family duties can be answered in this way—the family duties exist so long as one is in the ordinary consciousness. . . if the call to a spiritual life comes, whether one keeps to them or not depends partly upon the way of Yoga one follows, partly on one's own spiritual necessity. There are many who pursue inwardly the spiritual life and keep the family duties, not as social duties but as a field for the practice of *Karma Yoga*, others abandon everything to follow the spiritual call or line and they are justified if that is necessary for the Yoga they practise or if that is the imperative demand of the soul within them."[1]

Again he writes: " 'Dedication of life' is quite possible for some without their staying here. It is a question of inward attitude and of the total consecration of the being

[1] *Letters*, Vol. IV, pp. 56-7.

to the Divine."[1] Elsewhere he remarks: "It is not absolutely necessary to abandon the ordinary life in order to
seek after the Light or to practise Yoga . . . it is only
necessary when the pressure of the inner urge becomes so
great that the pursuit of the ordinary life is no longer
compatible with the pursuit of the dominant spiritual
objective. Till then what is necessary is a power to practise
an inner isolation, to be able to retire within oneself and
concentrate at any time on the necessary spiritual purpose. There must also be a power to deal with the
ordinary outer life from a new attitude and one can
then make the happenings of that life itself a means for
the inner change of nature and the growth in spiritual
experience."[2]

Everyone is not so circumstanced, he observes, "that
they can cut loose from the ordinary life; they accept it
therefore as a field of experience and self-training in the
earlier stages of the sadhana. But they must take care to
look at it as a field of experience only and to get free from
the ordinary desires, attachments and ideas which usually
go with it, otherwise it becomes a drag and hindrance on
their sadhana."[3]

The best way to live "in the ordinary occupations and
surroundings is to cultivate an entire equality and detachment and the samata (equability) of the Gita with the
faith that the Divine is there and the Divine Will at work
in all things even though at present under the conditions
of a world of Ignorance".[4]

To the Western mind, with its emphasis on action and
its love of the actual and concrete, its longing for 'results'
it can see and analyse, Integral Yoga would be much
easier to appreciate if it were a system concerned with set

[1] *Letters*, Vol. II, p. 487.
[2] Ibid., pp. 481-2.
[3] Ibid.
[4] *More Lights on Yoga*, pp. 47-8.

postures, *prāṇāyāma* (control of the breath or vital power),
fixed meditation and so on—any outward observance
which would enable it to imagine with relief that it had
got 'something to catch hold of'. But instead of outward
asceticism it is offered inward askesis, "an inner discipline
far more exacting and difficult than mere ethical and
physical austerities".[1]

The characteristic reaction of the Westerner to this
intensive concentration on a complex inner world is often
to feel that he has, not something, but nothing to catch
hold of, that everything is slightly insubstantial, impre-
cise; that he has no way of taking accurate bearings. To
some extent this bias is probably present in most Western
aspirants, since they are normally more extroverted than
their Eastern fellows: where it is very intensely felt it may
indicate that this particular Yoga is not the right one for
the aspirant. It is well in this context to remember the
place given to work and action in the *sadhana* and to bear
in mind these words of Sri Aurobindo: "Those who have
an expansive creative vital or a vital made for action are
usually at their best when the vital is not held back from
its movements and they can develop faster by it than by
instrospective meditation. All that is needed is that the
action should be dedicated. . . . It is a mistake to think
that to live in introspective meditation all the time is invariably the best or the only way of Yoga."[2]

Although asceticism for its own sake is not part of
Integral Yoga, there are, however, certain simple practical observances connected with day-to-day living which
are essential to health and to the right conduct of the
sadhana, "for self-control in the vital (being) and right

---

[1] *Lights on Yoga*, p. 3. The ignorant adoption of postures, exercises,
etc., by the uninstructed has probably done more to discredit Yoga in
the West than anything else. In fact, the higher Yogas do not concern
themselves with these things.
[2] *Letters*, Vol. IV, pp. 605-6.

order in the material are a very important part of it (sadhana)".[1]

Sufficient food and sleep are necessary and Sri Aurobindo often quotes the *Gita's* injunction : "Yoga is not for one who eats too much or sleeps too much, neither is it for one who does not eat or does not sleep."[2] In this respect, *sadhakas* would seem to be divided into those who find it hard to cope with food-desire, and those who wish to stop eating and sleeping altogether! But here again, the emphasis is on moderation and right use, not on renunciation or repression.

A vegetarian diet makes the control of the vital nature easier, as well as being based "on a will not to do harm to the more conscious forms of life for the satisfaction of the belly".[3] Just as too much eating makes the body "material and heavy, eating too little makes it weak and nervous— one has to find the true harmony and balance between the body's need and the food taken".[4]

Equanimity and non-attachment are the way to deal with greed or vital desire in this Yoga, not fasting. Fasting, by increasing the vital energy beyond the nervous system's power to assimilate or co-ordinate, may produce a morbid condition in the body:[5] nervous people particularly "should avoid the temptation to fast, it is often

[1] *Bases of Yoga*, p. 77.
[2] *Letters*, Vol. II, p. 427.
[3] Ibid., p. 426.
[4] *Letters*, Vol. IV, p. 553.
[5] "A premature and excessive physical austerity, Tapasya, may endanger the process of the sadhana by establishing a disturbance and abnormality of the forces in the different parts of the system. A great energy may pour into the mental and vital parts, but the nerves and the body may be overstrained and lose strength to support the play of these higher energies. This is the reason why an extreme physical austerity is not included here as a substantive part of the sadhana.
There is no harm in fasting from time to time for a day or two or in reducing the food taken to a small but sufficient modicum; but entire abstinence for a long period is not advisable." (*Bases of Yoga*, p. 82.)

accompanied or followed by delusions and a loss of balance".[1] "Such fasting is frequently suggested by the vital Entities, because it puts the consciousness into an unbalanced state which favours their designs. It is therefore discouraged here."[2]

The question of sleep, of dreams, of the various inner worlds into which people penetrate in sleep and of their relevance to spiritual development, is a very great one and is dealt with at length by Sri Aurobindo in his *Letters* and other books on Yoga. It is not possible to do more than indicate it here, since it is too complex a subject to lend itself easily to simplification. It is, however, worth noting that the ability to become conscious in sleep marks a high advance and is a necessary part of the integrating process of the Yoga.

[1] *Letters*, Vol. IV, p. 81.
[2] Ibid., p. 46.

CHAPTER VII

THE DIVINE PRESENCE

> Live always as if you were under the very eye of the
> Supreme.
>
> *More Lights on Yoga*, p. 80.

IT WOULD be impossible in an introduction to Integral
Yoga, such as this attempts to be, to touch-in more than
the salient points in its practice and to indicate some of
the problems the aspirant may encounter in his development.

The endeavour that Yoga—and particularly this Yoga
—sets before the *sadhaka* is an immense one, full of difficulties and dangers and problems of personal application,
far too many in number for anyone to do more than
indicate in a limited way in a small book. Were it not so,
Sri Aurobindo presumably would not have found it necessary, in exposition of his spiritual philosophy and Yoga,
to produce sufficient material to fill over twenty books.

The core of the Mystery, when we reach it, may be of
the most crystalline simplicity, but its attainment requires for most of us an exercise of the utmost complexity,
since it is essentially one of disentanglement. Indeed, one
of the worst mistakes we may make is to over-simplify
the problems that confront us before we have achieved
that condition of simplicity when problems cease to be
central, and imagine in our haste, impatience or defiance
that we can hack our way violently to the centre, anni-
hilating the powers of our being as we go, instead of
patiently unwinding the veils from the Mystery one by
one. Those who try rashly to take the Kingdom of Heaven
by storm, says Sri Aurobindo, are in for a rough time.

As we mentioned in the chapter on 'Surrender', there
are three processes in the spiritual movement towards
union with God: firstly, the act of self-consecration or
surrender to the Divine, fairly easy to initiate but extremely difficult to execute fully; secondly, a standing
apart from the *adhara* through self-knowledge so that the
soul ceases to identify itself with the outer nature; and
thirdly, "the vision of God everywhere in all things and
in all happenings, the surrender of the fruits of action and
action itself to God, and the freedom thereby from ignorance, from egoism, from duality, from desire".[1] Then it
can be said of God: "All that is, is he and he is More than
all that is." To become aware of this truth, to realize it
and make it effective, whether it comes by knowledge,
works, love or any other means, is, says Sri Aurobindo,
the object of all Yoga.

Long before we have anything but an intellectual
inkling of what this realization implies, we can perhaps
dimly apprehend a little of its state through such potent
sayings as: "In that Light shall ye see light," and not
only catch from time to time small flashes of our own of
its wonder, but see in truly God-realized men, like Aurobindo, something of what its possession means. But
though such an experience, as an abiding condition of our
consciousness, lies at the summit of the Yoga, the guidance
of the Divine in the *sadhana* is not dependent on its
attainment and may be realized before the preparation of
the nature has been finished, provided there is "trust and
confidence in the Divine and the will to surrender".

Such a taking up of the *sadhana* by the Divine,[2] says
Sri Aurobindo, involves not only this perfect trust and

[1] *The Yoga and its Objects*, p. 44.
[2] Descent and transformation in fact depend on an increasing contact and union with the Divine, who gives the fruit, Sri Aurobindo
writes, not by the measure of the sadhana, but by the measure of the
soul's sincerity and aspiration.

confidence in Him and a progressive self-giving; it also involves putting oneself into His hands and ceasing to rely on one's own efforts alone. "It is in fact the principle of sadhana that I myself followed and it is the central process of the Yoga as I envisage it. . . . But all cannot follow that at once; it takes time for them to arrive at it —it grows most when the mind and vital (being) fall quiet."[1]

This surrender is an inner surrender of the mind and vital being and an outer surrender in which everything is given up that is found to conflict with the spirit or needs of the *sadhana*, "the offering, the obedience to the guidance of the Divine, whether directly, if one has reached that stage, or through the psychic (being) or to the guidance of the Guru".[2] He emphasizes in many places that the core of the inner surrender is trust and confidence in the Divine, which leads to a perfect self-giving. Into that attitude the aspirant must grow, and provided the will for it is maintained, grow he, or she, will; the rest is a matter of obedience to the guidance when it makes itself manifest, and of not allowing vital or mental movements to interfere.

He adds, however, that this is not the only way that *sadhana* can be done; there are many other ways by which the Divine can be approached. "But this is the only one I know by which the taking up of the sadhana by the Divine becomes a sensible fact before the preparation of the nature is done. . . . The idea and experience of the Divine doing all belong to the Yoga based on surrender. But whatever way is followed, the one thing to be done is to be faithful and go on to the end."[3]

We have already dealt with the important place given to the guidance of the soul, or psychic being, in this Yoga,

[1] *Letters*, Vol. I, p. 77.
[2] Ibid, pp. 77-8
[3] Ibid, p. 79.

which is based on the heart, the deepest, as the mind is the widest, power of consciousness. The soul as a projection of the Self is closely linked with the Divine—it is, indeed a spark of the Divine—and can give unfaltering guidance in the *sadhana*. But its full appearance and mastery take time to develop and belong, as does the guidance of the Divine, to mature stages of the Yoga. The aspirant must therefore rely on the Teacher, the Master or *Guru*, in the beginning; that is, on one who has already travelled the path and attained to mastery in it.

The control and discipline of the *Guru* is indispensable in the early stages, according to Sri Aurobindo. "All true Gurus are the same, the one Guru, because all are the Divine," he writes on this point. "That is a fundamental and universal truth. But there is also a truth of difference; the Divine dwells in different personalities with different minds, teachings, influences so that he may lead different disciples with their special need, character, destiny by different ways to the realization. Because all Gurus are the same Divine, it does not follow that the disciple does well if he leaves the one meant for him to follow another. Fidelity to the Guru is demanded of every disciple, according to the Indian tradition."[1]

The *Guru* must have the knowledge and know the way. He may have human defects and deficiencies. He may not even have the spiritual potentialities of the disciple he teaches, but provided the disciple sees in him the Grace of the Divine and opens himself to that, none of these things matter.

"It is not the human defects of the Guru that can stand in the way when there is the psychic opening, confidence and surrender. The Guru is the channel or the representative of the manifestation of the Divine, according to the measure of his personality or his attainment; but whatever he is, it is to the divine that one opens in

[1] *Letters*, Vol. II, pp. 267-8.

opening to him; and if something is determined by the power of the channel, more is determined by the inherent and intrinsic attitude of the receiving consciousness, an element that comes out in the surface mind as simple trust or direct unconditional self-giving, and once that is there, the essential things can be gained even from one who seems to others than the disciple an inferior spiritual source, and the rest will grow up in the sadhak of itself by the Grace of the divine, even if the human being in the Guru cannot give it."[1]

In difficult phases where the personal effort of the aspirant is frustrated, the *Guru* can intervene to bring about what is needed. In those periods of discouragement, particularly dangerous for the novice (for it is possible then to fall for good), the support of the *Guru* may help conclusively to steady a wavering faith and in all ways his knowledge and experience are of inestimable value.

Sri Aurobindo has pointed out that if one learns all by oneself the chances are that one will learn all wrong. Nevertheless, he qualifies this observation elsewhere by saying that the actual relationship of *Guru* and disciple is only one of many relations which the seeker may have with the Divine. As long as the soul needs it, it can be kept, but it must not be so bound by it that it closes itself to the inflow of any other relations it may have with the Supreme. The Buddha's remark, when he likened his teaching to a raft which a man does not need to carry on his head, once he has crossed the river, aptly illustrates the need to be aware of subtle spiritual attachments.

In the West we are denied the inestimable advantage of contact with individuals who embody what we are striving to attain ourselves. Though we undoubtedly produce from time to time individuals of outstanding moral stature and even of great sanctity, we simply do not now possess men, or women, who have attained realization or en-

---

[1] *Letters*, Vol. II, p. 271.

lightenment in the sense in which these terms are meant in the East. However, the 'force' of a great Yogi is not limited by physical location and can act, as Sri Aurobindo has himself stated, on individuals many thousands of miles away. Given the right conditions of receptivity and faith a 'call' made in danger and difficulty will always bring a response.

As we have seen, Integral Yoga aims at the realization of the Divine Presence taking up the Yoga directly, not acting from behind in a veiled capacity, as in the beginning, and this, Sri Aurobindo states, is a greater and more intimate relation than that of the human *Guru* and disciple, which is more of a limited mental ideal.

By prayer, aspiration and surrender, and by an inner condition of openness, the aspirant calls to the Divine for help, and whether the response is felt or not, it is the Divine Force that is at work in the *sadhana* from the first, though it may have to work deeply, secretly and invisibly, in a way hidden from the ordinary surface nature. "Be strong," says Sri Aurobindo, "in the faith that whatever is right and necessary will inevitably happen, even if it is not the result that you preferred or expected."[1] If you stumble, it is right for you to stumble at that moment. Learn by detachment and self-knowledge to watch the Divine working. "That God himself is the Guru, you will find when the knowledge comes to you; you will see how every little circumstance within you and without you has been subtly planned and brought about by infinite wisdom to carry out the natural process of the Yoga, how the internal and external movements are arranged and brought together to work on each other, so as to work out the imperfection and work in the perfection. An almighty love and wisdom are at work for your uplifting. Therefore never be troubled by the time that is being taken, even if it seems very long."[2]

[1] *The Yoga and its Objects*, p. 24.
[2] Ibid., pp. 47-8.

This consciousness of the Divine Power at work in the *sadhana* clearly comes to people in insights of varying kinds. To some, as Sri Aurobindo describes in this passage, it may be through a gradual perception of the profound significance and rightness of all experience, calling not for a blind or stoical acceptance, though that may serve in the beginning, but to a spiritually creative meeting of its tests and challenges. Others may feel it as a descent of peace, light or power, or as a calm certainty of the Divine Force working in the *sadhana* through inward pressure or direction. The sense of peace in mind, life, body and surrounding the individual everywhere is, as we mentioned elsewhere, a sure sign of the Divine's presence. If you feel this consciousness, says Sri Aurobindo, call it in more and more to govern your effort and to take it up. There will then be a progressive transfer of the forces at work in the *adhara*. Until this is complete there must be what he calls the psychic poise, which discriminates carefully between the Divine Force, the element of personal effort, and what is brought in as a mixture from the lower cosmic forces.

While the transfer is still continuing, there must always be a personal contribution which rejects any lower mixture and assents only to the true Force. Even when the psychic being is in front and the work of the *sadhana* can be left in the hands of the Divine, constant vigilance is still required.

To those who have not yet achieved consciousness of the Divine influence, he advises that they should have faith and aspire for the opening. Surrender is the best way of opening, but aspiration and quietness can do it up to a certain point, lacking surrender. He gives also three necessary conditions for receiving the Divine Power and enabling it to act through the aspirant in the outward life. These are:

(i) Quietude, equality—not to be disturbed by anything that happens, to keep the mind still and firm, seeing the play of forces, but itself tranquil.

(ii) Absolute faith—faith that what is for the best will happen, but also that if one can make oneself a true instrument, the fruit will be that which one's will guided by the Divine Light sees as the thing to be done—*kartavyam karma*.[1]

(iii) Receptivity—the power to receive the Divine Force and to feel its presence and the presence of the Mother in it and allow it to work, guiding one's sight and will and action. If this power and presence can be felt and this plasticity made the habit of the consciousness in action—but this plasticity to the Divine Force alone without bringing in any foreign element—the eventual result is sure.[2]

Once the peace has been established, the Force can descend from above and work in the *adhara* more directly. It usually descends, we are told, first of all into the head, liberating the inner mind-centres, then into the heart-centre, liberating fully the psychic and emotional being, then into the navel and other vital centres, liberating the inner vital being, and lastly into the *muladhara* (base of spine), liberating the inner physical being. It works at the same time for perfection as well as liberation, taking up the whole nature, part by part. "It integrates, harmonizes, establishes a new rhythm in the nature. It can bring down, too, a higher and yet higher force and range of the higher nature until, if that be the aim of the sadhana, it becomes possible to bring down the supramental force and existence."[3]

In this process of the descent and its working, Sri Aurobindo adds warningly, it is vital to rely on the guidance of the *Guru* and not on one's own judgement.

---

[1] *Kartavyam karma*: duty.
[2] *Bases of Yoga*, pp. 18-19.
[3] *Lights on Yoga*, p. 38.

The forces of the lower nature may become excited and mix with the descent; undivine Powers may masquerade as the Divine and claim the *sadhaka's* service.

"If these things are accepted," he writes, "there will be an extremely disastrous consequence. If indeed there is the assent of the sadhak to the Divine working alone and the submission or surrender to that guidance, then all can go smoothly. This assent and a rejection of all egoistic forces or forces that appeal to the ego are the safeguard throughout the sadhana. But the ways of nature are full of snares, the disguises of the ego are innumerable, the illusions of the Powers of darkness are extraordinarily skilful; the reason is an insufficient guide and often turns traitor; vital desire is always with us tempting to follow any alluring call. This is the reason why we insist in this Yoga so much on what we call samarpana—rather inadequately rendered by the English word surrender. If the heart-centre is fully opened and the psychic (being) is always in control, then there is no question; all is safe. But the psychic can at any moment be veiled by a lower upsurge. . . . The guidance of one who himself is by identity or represents himself as the Divine is in this difficult endeavour imperative and indispensable."[1]

To the beginner, trying laboriously to turn the precept of *samarpana* into practice, however haltingly, things like the descent of the Truth-Consciousness and the dynamic realization of God in all things and happenings, which are the crown of the Yoga, may seem as remote and unattainable as the ascent of Everest to someone whose capacities have been fully exercised in panting to the top of Ben Nevis.

The aspirant knows that there are those who have won the crown, and though he may (and must) fix his eyes on them in faith and confidence as the guarantors of his own eventual attainment, however long-delayed and seemingly

[1] *Lights on Yoga*, pp. 41-2.

impossible, he is all too apt, in moments of reversal, to think that they were all beings of extraordinary spiritual ability and to forget that the operative factor in their attainment was the Divine Grace, which is there for all who can open to it.

At these moments of despondency, says Sri Aurobindo, remember two things: that there is only one truth in you on which you must lay constant hold, the truth of your divine potentialities; and secondly, the call of the Light to your nature. If you cling firmly to this, or, if you are shaken from your hold, return to it constantly, it will justify itself in the end in spite of all stumblings and obstacles. If you have chosen the Divine, you can be certain that the Divine first chose you.

Take with you the peace and quietude and joy and keep it by remembering always the Divine.

More Lights on Yoga, p. 55.

APPENDIX

SRI AUROBINDO on *The Spiritual Man* and *The Divine Life*: a selection taken from his writings:

The Master and Mover of our works is the One, the Universal and Supreme, the Eternal and Infinite. . . . All that is is he, and he is the More than all that is, and we ourselves, though we know it not, are being of his being, force of his force, conscious with a consciousness derived from his; even our mortal existence is made out of his substance and there is an immortal within us that is a spark of the Light and Bliss that are for ever. No matter whether by knowledge, works, love or any other means, to become aware of this truth of our being, to realize it, to make it effective here or elsewhere is the object of all Yoga.
The Synthesis of Yoga, p. 241.

The perfect supramental action will not follow any single principle or limited will. It is not likely to satisfy the standard either of the individual egoist or of any organized group-mind. It will conform to the demand neither of the positive practical man of the world nor of the formal moralist nor of the patriot nor of the sentimental philanthropist nor of the idealizing philosopher. It will proceed by a spontaneous outflowing from the summits in the totality of an illumined and uplifted being, will and knowledge and not by the selected, calculated and standardized action which is all that the intellectual reason or ethical will can achieve. Its sole aim will be the expression of the divine within us and the keeping together of the world and its progress towards the Manifestation that is to be. This even will not be so much an aim and purpose as a spontaneous law of the being and an intuitive
163

determination of the action by the Light of the divine Truth and its automatic influence. It will proceed like the action of nature from a total will and knowledge behind her, but a will and knowledge enlightened in a conscious supreme Nature and no longer obscure in this ignorant Prakriti. It will be an action not bound by the dualities but full and large in the spirit's impartial joy of existence. The happy and inspired movement of a divine Power and Wisdom guiding and impelling us will replace the perplexities and stumblings of the suffering and ignorant ego.

If by some miracle of divine intervention all mankind at once could be raised to this level, we should have something on earth like the Golden Age of the traditions, Satya Yuga, the Age of Truth or true existence. For the sign of the Satya Yuga is that the Law is spontaneous and conscious in each creature and does its own works in a perfect harmony and freedom. Unity and universality, not separative division, would be the foundation of the consciousness of the race; love would be absolute; equality would be consistent with hierarchy and perfect in difference; absolute justice would be secured by the spontaneous action of the being in harmony with the truth of things and the truth of himself and others and therefore sure of the truth and right result; right reason, no longer mental but supramental, would be satisfied not by the observation of artificial standards but by the free automatic perception of right relations and their inevitable execution in the act. The quarrel between the individual and society or disastrous struggle between one community and another could not exist: the cosmic consciousness imbedded in embodied beings would assure a harmonious diversity in oneness.

Ibid., pp. 194–5.

Let us not be in too furious a haste to acquire even peace, purity and perfection. Peace must be ours, but not the peace of an empty or devastated nature or of slain or mutilated capacities incapable of unrest because we have made them incapable of intensity and fire and force. Purity must be our aim, but not the purity of a void or of a bleak and rigid coldness. Perfection is demanded of us, but not the perfection that can exist only by confining its scope within narrow limits or putting an arbitrary full stop to the ever self-extending scrolls of the Infinite. Our object is to change into the divine nature, but the divine nature is not a mental or moral but a spiritual condition, difficult to achieve, difficult even to conceive by our intelligence. The Master of our work and our Yoga knows the thing to be done, and we must allow him to do it in us by his own means and in his own manner. . . . It is easier to starve the ego by renouncing the impulse to act or to kill it by cutting away from us all the movement of personality. It is easier to exalt it into self-forgetfulness immersed in a trance of peace or an ecstasy of divine Love. But our more difficult problem is to liberate the true Person and attain to a divine manhood which shall be the pure vessel of a divine force and the perfect instrument of a divine action.

Ibid., pp. 245–6.

A Yoga turned towards an all-embracing realization of the Supreme will not despise the works or even the dreams, if dreams they are, of the Cosmic Spirit or shrink from the splendid toil and many-sided victory which he has assigned to himself in the human creature. But its first condition for this liberality is that our works in the world, too, must be part of the sacrifice offered to the Highest and none else, to the Divine Shakti and to no other Power, in the right spirit and with the right knowledge, by the free soul and not by the hypnotized bond-slave of material Nature. . . . All activities of knowledge that seek after or express Truth are in themselves rightful

materials for a complete offering; none ought necessarily
to be excluded from the wide framework of the divine life.
The mental and physical sciences which examine into the
laws and forms and processes of things, those which concern the life of men and animals, the social, political,
linguistic and historical and those which seek to know and
control the labours and activities by which man subdues
and utilizes his world and environment, and the noble and
beautiful Arts which are at once work and knowledge—
for every well-made and significant poem, picture, statue
or building is an act of creative knowledge, a living discovery of the consciousness, a figure of Truth, a dynamic
form of mental and vital self-expression or world-expres-
sion—all that seeks, all that finds, all that voices or figures
is a realization of something of the play of the Infinite and
to that extent can be made a means of God-realization or
of divine formation. But the Yogin has to see that it is
no longer done as part of an ignorant mental life; it can
be accepted by him only if by the feeling, the remembrance, the dedication within it, it is turned into a movement of the spiritual consciousness and becomes a part of
its vast grasp of comprehensive illuminating knowledge.
                                        Ibid., pp. 112–13.

The spiritual or supramental Self, the Divine Being,
the supreme and immanent Reality, must be alone the
Lord within us and shape freely our final development
according to the highest, widest, most integral expression
possible of the law of our nature. In the end that nature
acts in the perfect Truth and its spontaneous freedom; for
it obeys only the luminous power of the Eternal. The
individual has nothing further to gain, no desire to fulfil;
he has become a portion of the impersonality or the
universal personality of the Eternal. No other object than
the manifestation and play of the Divine Spirit in life and
the maintenance and conduct of the world in its march

towards the divine goal can move him to action. Mental ideas, opinions, constructions are his no more; for his mind has fallen into silence, it is only a channel for the Light and Truth of the divine knowledge. Ideals are too narrow for the vastness of his spirit; it is the ocean of the Infinite that flows through him and moves him for ever.

Ibid., pp. 198–9.

For, even after he is free, the sadhaka will be in the world and to be in the world is to remain in works. But to remain in works without desire is to act for the good of the world in general or for the kind or the race or for some new creation to be evolved on the earth or some work imposed by the Divine Will within him. And this must be done either in the framework provided by the environment or the grouping in which he is born or placed or else in one which is chosen or created for him by a divine direction. Therefore in our perfection there must be nothing left in the mental being which conflicts with or prevents our sympathy and free self-identification with the kind, the group or whatever collective expression of the Divine he is meant to lead, help or serve. But in the end it must become a free self-identification through identity with the Divine and not a mental bond or moral tie of union or a vital association dominated by any kind of personal, social, national, communal or credal egoism.

Ibid., p. 201.

In an advanced stage of the Yoga it is indifferent to the seeker, in the sense of any personal preference, what action he shall do or not do; even whether he shall act or not is not decided by his personal choice or preference. Always he is moved to do whatever is in consonance with the Truth or whatever the Divine demands through his nature. . . . After liberation a man may dwell in any sphere

of life and in any kind of action and fulfil there his existence in the Divine. . . . If such be the intention of the
Supreme within him, the liberated soul may be content
with a subtle and limited action within the old human
surroundings which will in no way seek to change their
outward appearance. But it may, too, be called to a work
which will not only alter the forms and sphere of its own
external life but, leaving nothing around it unchanged or
unaffected, create a new world or a new order.

Ibid., pp. 272–3.

The true salvation or the true freedom from the chain
of rebirth is not the rejection of terrestrial life or the
individual's escape by a spiritual self-annihilation, even
as the true renunciation is not the mere physical abandonment of family and society; it is the inner identification
with the Divine in whom there is no limitation of past life
and future birth but instead the eternal existence of the
unborn Soul. . . . It is immaterial whether he (the liberated
soul) wears the garb of an ascetic or lives the full life of the
householder; whether he spends his days in what men call
holy works or in the many-sided activities of the world;
whether he devotes himself to the direct leading of men to
the Light like Buddha, Christ or Shankara or governs
kingdoms like Janaka or stands before men like Sri
Krishna as a politician or a leader of armies; what he
eats or drinks; what are his habits or pursuits; whether
he fails or succeeds; whether his work be one of construction or destruction; whether he supports or restores an
old order or labours to replace it by a new. . . . He is not
governed by the judgements of men or the laws laid down
by the ignorant; he obeys an inner voice and is moved by
an unseen Power. His real life is within and this is its
description that he lives, moves and acts in God, in the
Divine, in the Infinite.

Ibid., pp. 276–8.

The liberated man has no personal hopes; he does not seize on things as his personal possessions; he receives what the divine Will brings him, covets nothing, is jealous of none: what comes to him he takes without repulsion and without attachment; what goes from him he allows to depart into the whirl of things without repining or grief or sense of loss. His heart and self are under perfect control; they are free from reaction and passion, they make no turbulent response to the touches of outward things.

Essays on the Gita (First Series), p. 249.

The Divine, the Eternal, expresses himself as existence, consciousness, bliss, wisdom, knowledge, love, beauty, and we can think of him as these impersonal and universal powers of himself, regard them as the nature of the Divine and Eternal; we can say that God is Love, God is Wisdom, God is Truth or Righteousness: but he is not himself an impersonal state or abstract of states or qualities; he is the Being, at once absolute, universal and individual. If we look at it from this basis, there is, very clearly, no opposition, no incompatibility, no impossibility of a co-existence or one-existence of the Impersonal and the Person; they are each other, live in one another, melt into each other and yet in a way can appear as if different ends, sides, obverse and reverse of the same Reality. The gnostic being is of the nature of the Divine and therefore repeats in himself this natural mystery of existence.

The Life Divine, Vol. II (2), p. 1069.

This, then, would be the nature of the gnostic Person, an infinite and universal being revealing—or, to our mental ignorance, suggesting—its eternal self through the significant form and expressive power of an individual and temporal self-manifestation.

Ibid., p. 1072.

A gnostic collectivity would be a collective soul-power of the Truth-consciousness, even as the gnostic individual would be an individual soul-power of it: it would have the same integration of life and action in unison, the same realized and conscious unity of being, the same spontaneity, intimate oneness-feeling, one and mutual truth-vision and truth-sense of self and each other, the same truth-action in the relation of each with each and all with all; this collectivity would be and act not as a mechanical but a spiritual integer. A similar inevitability of the union of freedom and order would be the law of the collective life; it would be a freedom of the diverse play of the Infinite in divine souls. . . . The greatest richness of diversity in the self-expression of the one-ness would be the law of the gnostic life. In the gnostic consciousness difference would not lead to discord but to a spontaneous natural adaptation, a sense of complementary plenitude, a rich many-sided execution of the thing to be collectively known, done, worked out in life.

Ibid., pp. 1094-5.

In the gnostic or divine being, in the gnostic life, there will be a close and complete consciousness of the self of others, a consciousness of their mind, life, physical being which are felt as if they were one's own. The gnostic being will act, not out of a surface sentiment of love and sympathy or any similar feeling, but out of this close mutual consciousness, this intimate oneness. All his action in the world will be enlightened by a truth of vision of what has to be done, a sense of the will of the Divine Reality in him which is also the Divine Reality in others. . . .

It is, then, this spiritual fulfilment of the urge to individual perfection and an inner completeness of being that we mean first when we speak of a divine life. It is the first essential condition of a perfected life on earth, and we are therefore right in making the utmost possible

individual perfection our first supreme business. The perfection of the spiritual and pragmatic relation of the individual with all around him is our second preoccupation;
the solution of this second desideratum lies in a complete
universality and oneness with all life upon earth which is
the other concomitant result of an evolution into the
gnostic consciousness and nature. But there still remains
the third desideratum, a new world, a change in the total
life of humanity or, at the least, a new perfected collective
life in the earth-nature. This calls for the appearance not
only of isolated evolved individuals acting in the un-
evolved mass, but of many gnostic individuals forming a
new kind of beings and a new common life superior to the
present individual and common existence.

Ibid., pp. 1124–6.

The one rule of the gnostic life would be the self-
expression of the Spirit, the will of the Divine Being; that
will, that self-expression could manifest through extreme
simplicity or through extreme complexity and opulence
or in their natural balance—for beauty and plenitude, a
hidden sweetness and laughter in things, a sunshine and
gladness of life are also powers and expressions of the
Spirit. In all directions the Spirit within determining the
law of the nature would determine the frame of the life
and its detail and circumstance. In all there would be the
same plastic principle; a rigid standardization, however
necessary for the mind's arrangement of things, could not
be the law of the spiritual life. A great diversity and
liberty of self-expression based on an underlying unity
might well become manifest; but everywhere there would
be harmony and truth of order.

Ibid., p. 1181.

Lastly, to be fully is to have the full delight of being.
Being without delight of being, without an entire delight

of itself and all things is something neutral or diminished; it is existence, but it is not fulness of being. This delight too, must be intrinsic, self-existent, automatic; it cannot be dependent on things outside itself: whatever it delights in, it makes part of itself, has the joy of it as part of its universality. . . . To become complete in being, in consciousness of being, in force of being, in delight of being and to live in this integrated completeness is the divine living.

Ibid., p. 1116.

adhara . .	.	the containing system of mind, life and body. It is composed of five sheaths, physical, vital, mental, supramental and spiritual.
advaita . .	.	vedantic.
ajnacakra .	.	see under *cakra*.
anahata . .	.	see under *cakra*.
ananda . .	.	bliss. It is the third term in the Hindu definition of the Godhead, *saccid-ananda*, Being-Consciousness-Bliss.
apramatta		without losing oneself.
asana . .	.	posture.
asubha . .	.	evil.
atman .	.	Self or Spirit: see under Self.
avatara (Avatar)	.	the descent of the Divine in human form.
bhakta . .	.	devotee, lover of the divine: hence *bhakti*, devotion.
cakra (Chakra) .	.	centre: the seven psychological centres in the subtle body.
—*ajna* .	.	forehead centre.
—*anahata* .	.	heart centre.
—*hrdpadma* .	.	heart lotus; the same as *anahata*.
—*manipura*	.	centre at navel.
—*muladhara*	.	centre at base of spine.
—*sahasradala*	.	overhead centre; 'thousand - petalled lotus'.
—*svadhisthana*	.	abdominal centre.
—*visuddha* .	.	throat centre.
Desire-soul .	.	ego.
dharma . .	.	the law of being.
Ego . .	.	the nexus of imperfect consciousness and knowledge gathered together in the being's push out of the Ignorance: the sense which makes man identify himself with the creation Nature has made of him.
guna . .	.	a mode or quality of Nature.
guru . .	.	spiritual master, teacher, one with knowledge of the Way, who embodies the Divine.

173

hrdpadma	. .	see under *cakra*.
japa	. . .	repetition of set sounds or words or a name as a prayer.
jnana	. . .	wisdom, knowledge.
karma	. . .	action, work; the resulting force of acts done in the past, particularly in past lives.
karma yoga	. .	a Yoga which takes work, dedicated to the Divine, as its basis.
kartavyam karma	.	duty.
lingha deha —*sarira*	. . }	subtle body.
mantra	. . .	set words or sounds having a spiritual significance or power.
mayavada	. .	the theory of Illusionism.
Mental being	. .	that part of the nature concerned with cognition, intelligence, ideas, mental or thought perceptions, mental vision, will, etc.
Mind	. . .	the centre of the (limited) functioning of consciousness of the mental being; its powers are those of delimitation, formal definition, analysis, division, discrimination.
moksa (*Moksha*)	.	liberation from illusion or unreality.
mukti	. . .	spiritual liberation.
muladhara	. .	see under *cakra*.
om .	. . .	the primal sound representing the supreme spiritual reality.
Overmind	. .	the principle linking mind with supermind.
prakrti (*Prakriti*)	.	Nature as active and executive energy.
prana	. . .	life.
pranayama	. .	control of the breath or vital power.
psychic	. . .	pertaining to the soul.
psychic being	. .	that part of the soul which supports the mind, vital sheath and physical body.
psychicisation	. .	the psychic transformation of the nature.
purusa (*Purusha*)	.	the soul: see also under soul.
rajas	. . .	one of the three *gunas* or fundamental modes of nature; the kinetic principle, defined psychologically as the active (rajasic) type of individual.
rsi (*Rishi*)	. .	Sage, Seer.

sadhaka . . .	one who practises a system of Yoga.
sadhana . . .	the practice of Yoga.
sakti (Shakti) . .	the divine cosmic energy, the power of the Infinite, the Divine Mother or Creatrix.
samadhi . . .	Yoga-trance; loss of consciousness of the outside world, entire inner withdrawal.
samarpana . .	entire surrender, self-giving.
samata . . .	equability.
samsara . . .	the phenomenal world, that which moves or changes always.
samskaras . .	fixed mental formations, impressions of past habits, experiences stored up in the subconscious parts. It may also mean a purifying rite.
Sankhyas . .	School of analytic thinkers.
sannyasi . . .	an ascetic.
sattva (Sattwa) . .	one of the three *gunas* or fundamental modes of Nature; the principle of equilibrium, light and harmony, defined psychologically as the contemplative (sattwic) mental type of individual.
satya yuga . .	the Age of Truth.
Self . . .	the Atman: the true being of the individual, realized as the *same* being in all and the Self in the cosmos.
siddhi . . .	realization; it may also be an occult power gained by Yoga.
Soul . . .	purusha: an aspect of the Self; a spark of the Divine which descends into the manifestation to support its evolution in the material world.
Spirit . . .	Atman: see under Self.
Subtle body . .	the subtle sheaths enclosing the physical body; called sometimes 'the aura' or 'the etheric'.
suksma sarira . *—deha* .	} the subtle body.
Supermind . .	the Truth-Consciousness of God; an intermediate functioning of consciousness between the Pure Being of God and the inferior functioning of consciousness represented by Mind.
Supramental . .	pertaining to the Supermind.

svadharma   .   .   self-law; the being's own essential law of
  (Swadharma)   action.
svadhisthana   .   .   see under cakra.
tamas   .   .   .   one of the three gunas or fundamental
                       modes of Nature; her principle of
                       obscurity and inertia, psychologically
                       defined as the ignorant, inert (tamasic)
                       type of individual.
tapasya   .   .   .   spiritual discipline or process.
vairagya   .   .   distaste for the world and life; turning
                       away of the mind from the objects of
                       its attachment.
veda   .   .   .   ancient Indian scripture.
visuddha .   .   .   see under cakra.
Vital sheath, .   .   that part of the adhara or containing
  body or being   system concerned with emotion, feel-
                       ing, desire, etc.
yoga   .   .   .   union with the Divine; the discipline by
                       which one enters into an inner and
                       higher consciousness.
yogin   .   .   .   the mystic, contemplative, one who prac-
                       tises Yoga.

Books Consulted:
BY SRI AUROBINDO:

The Life Divine (3 Vols.)   Lights on Life-Problems
Essays on the Gita (First Series)   Elements of Yoga
Essays on the Gita (Second Series)   The Riddle of this World
The Human Cycle   The Yoga and its Objects
The Problem of Rebirth   The Ideal of Human Unity
The Supramental Manifestation   Sri Aurobindo on himself and
The Mother   the Mother
Kena Upanishad   A Glossary of Sanskrit terms in
Eight Upanishads   the Life Divine
Hymns to the Mystic Fire
The Synthesis of Yoga   Sri Aurobindo, by G. H. Langley
Letters of Sri Aurobindo (4 Vols.)   Sri Aurobindo,
Bases of Yoga   by K. R. Srinivasa Iyengar
Lights on Yoga   The Philosophy of Integralism,
More Lights on Yoga   by Haridas Chaudhuri

The Dawn Horse Press is dedicated to the publication of classic spiritual literature, the work of authentic spiritual genius, from all traditions and times, through the present day. We are committed to the preparation of well-designed and yet reasonably priced editions, and we are determined to see that these books stay in print from generation to generation. We consider publishing to be a form of spiritual practice and service that promotes the great tradition of true knowledge and implements the growth of a genuine human intelligence in the world.

The Laughing Man Series of Classic Spiritual Literature is a selection of books representing various traditions in the spiritual heritage of mankind. This series is published in cooperation with The Laughing Man Institute for Traditional and Esoteric Studies, a non-profit organization devoted to examination of all paths, ancient and modern, that communicate the process of spiritual transformation.

THE DAWN HORSE PRESS

Other Publications from The Dawn Horse Press

The Dawn Horse Press makes available the Teaching of Bubba Free John through publication of works from The Free Communion Church.

THE KNEE OF LISTENING: *The Early Life and Radical Spiritual Teachings of Bubba Free John (Franklin Jones)* Foreword by Alan Watts
The first half of this book is an autobiographical account of Bubba's spiritual odyssey and a statement of his revelatory conclusions upon regaining Enlightenment. The second half communicates the essential wisdom of the radical Dharma of Understanding, which is a fulfillment and extension of all the Great Teachings of the past.

$3.95

THE METHOD OF THE SIDDHAS: *Talks with Bubba Free John (Franklin Jones) on the Spiritual Technique of the Saviors of Mankind*
In thirteen powerful talks given to his early devotees, Bubba Free John discourses on the means of implementing his Teaching. That means is the ancient one, Divine Communion, the transforming relationship between the devotee and the Perfect Spiritual Master, which matures as conscious Communion and, at last, radical Identity with God.

$3.95

GARBAGE AND THE GODDESS: *The Last Miracles and Final Spiritual Instructions of Bubba Free John*
An account of an intense and dramatic period of Bubba's Teaching work, which lasted from March until July, 1974. The talks published here are an extension and elaboration of his essential Teachings, and the narratives and personal accounts are a demonstration of that instruction in the very lives of his devotees.

$4.95

NO REMEDY: *An Introduction to the Life and Practices of The Free Communion Church, as Taught by Bubba Free John.*
Treating every aspect of spiritual life from diet to God-Realization, *No Remedy* provides a comprehensive picture of life in a true culture—The Free Communion Church—along with explicit instruction in its practices, by which individuals make the full transition from the suffering of common life to the sublime enjoyment of Only God.

$3.95

All available from The Free Communion Church, Star Route 2, Middletown, California 95461. Include $.35 per book for shipping. California residents add 6% tax.

Other books from
The Laughing Man Series

THE SONG OF THE SELF SUPREME (Astavakra Gita) Translated by Radhakamal Mukerjee
Few ancient treatises show such profound and lively concern with the ultimate reality. It presents Astavakra's teaching, based upon the Upanisadic creed of absolute monism, in the form of a dialogue with Janaka, the seer-king of Videha. This translation brings the true meaning of this illustrious Vedantic text to light for the first time for English readers and establishes it as one of the greatest texts in the history of spiritual literature.
$3.95

BREATH, SLEEP, THE HEART, AND LIFE: *The Revolutionary Health Yoga of Pundit Acharya* By Pundit Acharya.
Praised by the great Indian poet-mystic, Rabindranath Tagore, as well as by Western doctors and scientists, this delightful book shows the layman how to harmonize and spiritualize his life through simple and uniquely original exercises. The text is both practical and poetically graceful.
$3.95

THE YOGA OF LIGHT: *The Classic Esoteric Handbook of Kundalini Yoga* By Hans-Ulrich Reiker
Generally acknowledged as a classic, and translated with a wise and lively commentary by a modern practitioner, this traditional text gives the reader a step-by-step guide to the full realization of both hatha yoga (physical postures) and raja yoga ("the yoga of Light") as the single, integrated practice known and taught by the ancients.
$3.95

SAI BABA, THE SAINT OF SHIRDI By Mani Sahukar
Famous in India for his miracles, recognized by millions as a Divine incarnation, Sai Baba of Shirdi brought about a modern renaissance of the classic ancient path of devotion to the Spiritual Master. This account, devotional and yet scholarly, paints a vivid picture of this paradoxical, endearing saint.
$3.95

Available from The Dawn Horse Press, P.O. Box 677, Lower Lake, California, 95457. Include $.35 per book for shipping. California residents add 6% tax.